CALM UP

MINDFULNESS POCKETBOOK

First published in 2022 by Jake Mowbray.

© Jake Mowbray

A catalogue record for this book is available from the National Library of Australia at catalogue.nla.gov.au

Illustrations by Jules at Noonbit Studio
noonbitstudio.com / Instagram @noonbitstudio
Illustration art direction by Natalie Ex
natalieex.com / Instagram @natalie_ex

Cover & internal design and layout by Tess McCabe
tessmccabe.com.au

Edited & proofread by Amanda Druck
soothseeker.online

All web addresses are current at time of writing.

ISBN 9780646855035

Printed in Australia by Ingram Spark.

www.jakemowbraybooks.com
Instagram @jakemowbraybooks

DISCLAIMER
The views, opinions and thoughts expressed in this book belong solely to the author and are intended for the purpose of entertainment. This book should not be used as a substitute for professional assistance, therapeutic support or medical advice. In the event of physical or mental distress, please consult with appropriate health professionals. The application of ideas and information presented in this book are the choice of the reader, who assumes full responsibility for their understanding, interpretation or results. The author assumes no responsibility for the actions or choices of any reader.

CALM UP

MINDFULNESS POCKETBOOK

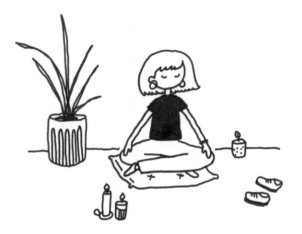

JAKE MOWBRAY

ILLUSTRATIONS BY JULES OF NOONBIT STUDIO

CONTENTS

Introduction   1

Balancing everything life has to throw at you   5

Meditation and breathing   29

Forgetting the past, not overthinking the future and being in the present   41

Introduction

I came across mindfulness when I was trying to find a way to not feel like shit all the time. A lot of us come to a point in our lives when we need to change something. For me, I would wake up with crippling anxiety in my chest every morning. This went on for five or so years before I finally thought, okay, something needs to be done here.

I have a stutter, which has led to many self-confidence issues and has amplified other insecurities in my life. Talking to strangers was terrifying. I would go out of my way to avoid any interaction with anyone I did not know on a deep level.

I went to the library for some inspiration and came across Eckhart Tolle's book, *The Power of Now*. After reading the first few pages, I was instantly hooked. Since then, I have implemented mindfulness into my daily life and now realise how powerful a tool it can be.

It is hard to be consistently happy every day. One day you wake up feeling a million bucks, the next day you may get up feeling angry, sad or anxious. Everyone gets this from time to time.

Trying to calm a racing mind can be difficult, especially if you are obsessing over the past or future, thinking about something somebody said, or angry at yourself for not going for a run (again).

The idea behind this book is to provide those who are going through a tough time something they can use to lift their mood, provide perspective to their thoughts or find techniques and strategies to help deal with a mental health issue they may be facing, all from the perspective of someone who is most likely just like you.

You can put this book in your work bag, keep it in the glove box of your car or pop it in your bedside drawer to pull out when you need it most. On the other hand, if you think it's all just a load of shit, put it in the bin — but please recycle.

You can read this book from start to finish, or you can just flick straight to a page that best reflects how you are feeling or go to a topic you would like to learn a little more about.

Like many other people, I have made mistakes. I have insecurities and regrets and will have more to deal with down the road. I wish I were able to say that this book is 100% a reflection of how my life is lived, but that would be far from the truth. I am still learning about myself and I am trying my best to improve each day.

Hopefully, by reading this book, you can turn tears into a smile, anxiety into motivation and sadness into optimism. Enjoy ☺

Notes and disclaimers

References and recommendations

We all stand on the shoulders of giants, and there are many great thinkers and public figures whose work and experiences I have drawn from and been inspired by in the writing of this book. However, it is important to me that this book should be easy to pick up and read, especially when you're feeling stressed – and making it look like a dense textbook wouldn't help with that much.

So, where it's relevant, I've mentioned sources, both academic and inspirational. At the end of some of the chapters, there's a section with recommendations of further reading, listening or viewing you might like to check. But the full details for all referenced works are available at the end of the book in the 'Referenced works and other recommendations' section if you would like to read further on any of the topics discussed in this book.

Qualifications, expertise and disclaimers

I just want to explicitly state that I am not an expert in any of the fields discussed in this book. I have no qualifications in any psychological fields at the time of writing this book. I have tried my best to gather knowledge from as many well-known professionals as I could find so you don't have to. If you are struggling with your mental health, please seek professional advice. The book is not intended to replace medical advice and should be used to supplement rather than replace regular care by your doctor or professional. It is recommended that you seek professional advice before embarking on any medical program or treatment. The publisher and author disclaim liability for any medical outcomes that may occur as a result of applying the methods suggested in this book.

Below are some sources you can use if you believe you need further help:

- Beyond Blue — 1300 22 46 36
- Black Dog Institute — www.blackdoginstitute.org.au
- Butterfly Foundation — 1800 33 4673
- Friendline — www.friendline.org.au
- Headspace — www.headspace.org.au
- Kids Help Line (can be used for people up to 25 years old) — 1800 55 18 00
- 1800RESPECT — 1800 737 732
- Parentline — 1300 1300 52
- Relationships Australia — 1300 364 277
- SANE Australia — 1800 187 263

BALANCING
EVERYTHING
LIFE HAS TO
THROW AT YOU

Evaluate what is important to you

Minimalism has become a trend in recent years. People are throwing out their clothes, their kitchen appliances, their furniture, their neighbours — okay, it may be a little too early for sarcasm. Whatever you throw out, the idea of this movement is to remove clutter to ensure sure you are only keeping the stuff you really need and use. This not only keeps living spaces clean and organised, but it can help keep your mind tidy, too.

If we start to implement this strategy into our lives, we will have better access to the things we often use, which will reduce the time it takes finding your things. Ultimately, this reduces stress levels as we are spending less time organising and taking care of items that add no value to our lives. Letting go of this stuff lifts a massive burden off our shoulders.

Minimalism can also be applied to the way we use our time. Being deliberate about where we allocate our time can be an effective tool to reduce the chances of wasting the day.

Planning does play a role in minimalism, but we need to make sure we are not *over*planning. Allow yourself breathing room for anything urgent or unexpected that may come up.

To become more minimalist with your time, start out by trying the following tips:

1. Set out three things you would love to become or do with your life.

2. When planning the details of how you'll spend your time, look to set short-term plans. This will allow your mind to focus on something that can be easily and quickly achieved.

3. When writing down how you'll spend your time, try to go for things that are essential to satisfy your

long-term aspirations. For example, if you are learning to play the piano, your long-term goal might be to go pro. You may set a short-term goal of spending 30 minutes a day learning a particular piece. By achieving your short-term goals, you are making small but positive steps towards your long-term goal.

4. If you realise you need to change your three things or adjust how you use your time, critically evaluate whether to 'keep or chuck' these aspirations and move on. A great strategy implemented by many people is the KonMari method made famous by Marie Kondo. KonMari is a simple process you can use to declutter your life — mainly through physical items. The method is based around one simple question: Does it bring you joy? When you are evaluating your three things, if something brings you joy you keep it. If you hesitate or say no, it's probably best to throw it out. It is as simple as that.

5. Focus on the journey of achieving your goals rather than the final destination. This can also apply to your mindfulness practice. As there is no ultimate state of mindfulness to be achieved, the focus should be on little improvements in one's awareness and mindset throughout their life's journey.

By prioritising what you want to focus your time on, you give yourself the freedom to direct your energy towards things you truly want to do; to use your time for the now.

You have a lot on your plate

'Being a person is hard.'

JERRY SEINFELD

You may hold a lot of different roles in your life: parent, partner, friend, employee, manager or entrepreneur. Managing these roles can be tough, especially when you are living a chaotic life.

Know your roles by writing them down, prioritising them and ensuring you are giving your time and energy towards the areas of your life that matter most.

As an example, let's take a look at a day in the life of uni student, Becky.

The table below gives an overview of the duties, roles and other commitments Becky has during her waking hours, from 6:30 am to 10:00 pm.

PRIORITY	ROLE	TIME SPENT TODAY	ACTIONED
1	Uni student	09:00–12:00	Went to a lecture and a tutorial. Did a bit of study at the library afterwards.
2	Daughter	19:00–20:00	Had dinner with family.
3	Friend	13:30–14:30	Met up with a friend for lunch.
4	Employee	15:00–18:00	Worked at the café.
5	Fitness/ active woman	07:00–08:00	Went for a run.
Spare Time		6.5 Hours	Used this time to commute, eat, catch up on further study and watched TV.

It's important to prioritise things in a way that will not bring on stress or anxiety, and that will allow us sufficient time to satisfy each of our important life roles. However, it is also important not to be overly strict with our regimes. This means allowing ourselves 'open' time that, if it is not put to a specific use, can be used as time to unwind. This is useful when something urgent comes up and we need to catch up on particular life commitments at a later date.

Let's say that just as Becky is about to go to sleep, she receives a message from one of her group assignment team members saying, 'Hey Bec, I still haven't finished my part coz I've been flat out at work. I know the assignment is due tomorrow and I'm so sorry. Would you be able to give me a hand?'

Becky decides to drop her morning run, as she sees this assignment as a priority over her fitness goals.

By organising our time in this way, the important people in our lives will appreciate the time we are putting towards them. Our friends feel like we want to be with them, our bosses know we are committed to the job, and our family can see that we care.

CHECK OUT

Stephen R. Covey, *The 7 Habits of Highly Effective People*.

Allocate time for you

'You can't stop the waves, but you can learn to surf.'
JON KABAT-ZINN, *Wherever You Go, There You Are*

If someone we love is sad, sick or going through a tough time, we tend to drop everything we're doing to look out for them. If we find ourselves in a dark place, do we always drop everything and look out for ourselves?

We spend most of our time at work, eating, and sleeping. Spend some time with yourself and write down how you are feeling. Are you anxious, depressed, happy, worn down, excited? It could be anything.

Once you have identified these emotions, describe why you feel this way. You could be worn down from work or feeling anxious due to a relationship with a lover.

By doing this we are able to identity these feelings and bring them to the surface. There is something about putting your emotions down on paper that makes these feelings less scary than they were at first.

It is also worth spending time alone. Depending on your lifestyle, you may be around people all the time. Take the time to isolate yourself from others and sit with your own thoughts. No phone, no Netflix—just you. You may do this through meditation or by lying in bed. You may want to focus on your breath, body, or just let your mind roam free without judgement or effort.

It would also be wise to pursue a hobby you love. We always make the excuse that we don't have time to do things we want to do. Take action. Make time. Give yourself as many opportunities to enjoy your life as possible.

These exercises will allow you to get more in touch with your emotions and improve your life, mentally and socially.

Never miss out on a full night's sleep

'Sleep is the single most effective thing we can do to reset our brain and body health each day — Mother Nature's best'

MATTHEW WALKER, *Why We Sleep*

Sleep may be one of the most vital and underappreciated health factors in our day-to-day lives. Many people find it difficult to get a full night's rest, whether due to mental health, physical health or the fact that, by the time they have finished everything for the day, they only have enough time to lie down for a few hours.

Most of us know we should be getting at least eight hours of sleep every night. In his book, *Why We Sleep*, neuroscientist and sleep researcher, Matthew Walker, states:

Humans need more than seven hours of sleep each night to maintain cognitive performance. After ten days of just seven hours of sleep, the brain is as dysfunctional as it would be after going without sleep for twenty-four hours.

If we are relying on coffee to get us through the day after having little sleep the night before, this will lead to growing mental health issues. We need to give our bodies a chance to recharge naturally. This may mean reducing the amount of caffeine you are consuming.

By getting a full night's rest on a regular basis, we are better able to manage our mental health and feel a lot more energised and alert when facing the day.

Some effective ways of improving your sleep are:

- No screens one hour before and after sleep. According to the National Sleep Foundation in the USA, 'the blue light emitted by screens on cell phones, computers, tablets, and televisions restrain the production of melatonin, the hormone that controls your sleep/wake cycle or circadian rhythm. Reducing melatonin makes it harder to fall and stay asleep'.

- Go to sleep and wake up at the same time every day. Routine is crucial for a good sleeping pattern, and inconsistency can lead to a rise in blood pressure.

- Sleep in the right environment. Make sure the room is dark and at a cool temperature.

- You can try to use sleep stories or meditation through an app or YouTube. There are plenty of them out there — experiment to find one that suits you.

- If you are finding it hard to sleep, get up and leave the room. Do something quiet and relaxing, such as reading a book, until you start to feel tired again.

We may spend hours every day doing it, but most of us are not experts on sleep. Matthew Walker is considered the guru on this topic. If you would like to read his work or watch him talk about the science and research behind how sleep affects us, I highly recommend you check out his book, *Why We Sleep*, or any of the many videos on YouTube in which he talks about his research.

CHECK OUT

Cleveland Clinic, 'Irregular sleep habits linked to poor health' (web article)

Matthew Walker, *Why We Sleep*

National Sleep Foundation, 'Three ways gadgets are keeping you awake' (web article).

Exercise, yoga and healthy eating

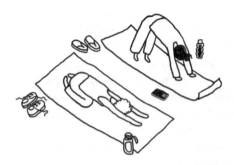

We all know that exercising regularly and watching what we eat are the two most important pillars of a healthy lifestyle, but actually committing to them can be seriously hard work. This is often why people resort to making poor food and lifestyle choices.

Healthy eating

We tend to snack while watching TV or working. It is often a comfort thing rather than a way to satisfy hunger. It is hard to be mindful of this when we are snacking on something we simply cannot resist — the last thing we want to do is stop.

Junk food and snacks are also seen to be a comfort mechanism for people who are going through a tough time. This is dangerous, as the dopamine rush we get from these foods gives us the false idea that these foods are going to make us feel better. They most certainly will not. This behaviour can often lead to junk food addictions as sugary and processed food forces the brain to create more dopamine receptors. People will often face withdrawals as they are craving a 'food high'. Healthy foods are just not as satisfying in that moment — you won't get the same dopamine high from eating an apple.

Minati Singh conducted a study in 2014 to identify how food intake is influenced by multiple factors, including mood and genes. The study showed:

> ... the influence of food choice includes biological determinants of hunger, appetite, and taste. Besides these, other factors of cost, income, and availability also influence food choice. Other determinants of social and psychological factors of mood, stress, and emotion also play a critical role in food choice.

It is hard to control certain environments in our life, however, by being more mindful of what we eat, we will find the ability to stop ourselves from demolishing a block of chocolate in one sitting. In turn, this will help us avoid the guilt and sugar hangover that inevitably comes afterwards. We can achieve this by strengthening our awareness and building good habits. Start to realise what foods are not going to be good for your body and look to take these foods out of your life. If your cupboard is filled with processed foods, return them to the shop or donate them to a food bank. If you are craving junk food, try to drink a glass of water or fill yourself up with more natural foods and see if your cravings are still present.

Other ways you can re-shape your eating life include:

- reducing portion sizes by using smaller plates or bowls

- taking and using a reusable water bottle wherever you go so you are always hydrated and will not resort to sugary drinks

- catch yourself out when you are mindlessly snacking or eating — look to be present in the moment when you are at the pantry or dinner table and avoid the triggers that can lead to unhealthy habits, such as snacking in front of the TV.

Yoga

Yoga has a lot of meditational properties. Known to be a great stress reliever, the practice also decreases anxiety, as your breathing brings awareness to particular body parts, shifting your attention away from any negative thoughts. It also can be an intense workout, if you choose to make it so, and can really strengthen your core and upper body by holding challenging body positions for extensive periods of time. Yoga, along with regular exercise, is a great way to stay in shape and calm your mind.

Exercise

Exercise can be a great way of releasing all the pent-up anger and anxiety we are holding within our bodies. You do not need to be Cadel Evans or LeBron James, as long as you are raising a bit of a sweat.

Try to push yourself a little more each time you exercise. For example, do a one kilometre run one day, try to run 1.5 kilometres the next time, and so on.

By doing regular exercise you are helping your mind clear negative and anxious thoughts. This will result in better sleep and improved relaxation. You will obviously start seeing great physical changes too.

Not sure where to begin? Start working on your exercise goals today with a quick circuit for beginners:

- 5 x push ups
- 10 x squats
- 30-second plank

- 10 x ab crunches
- 2-minute rest

Repeat this sequence four times.

This routine gives just a general idea of exercises you could do. If there are too many repetitions, lower it to two reps with a ten-second plank and work your way up. It is totally up to you. The key is to challenge your mind and body every day.

There will be days you really don't feel like doing exercise. The best advice we can give is to just start doing something. Whether that means driving to the gym, doing your first set of exercises or doing a warm-up. You may find if you just get started in this way, your exercises become less intimidating and you will begin your workout automatically.

CHECK OUT

Singh M. (2014). Mood, food, and obesity. *Frontiers in psychology*, 5, 925. https://doi.org/10.3389/fpsyg.2014.00925

Slow down, take a step back from life

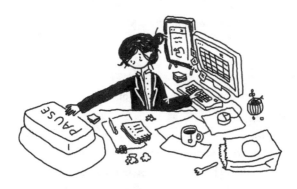

We are all trying to be the best version of ourselves. While working towards lofty goals, we can often end up getting caught up in the rat race of life — trying to get the perfect job, to get rich, find a spouse, keep everyone happy and so on.

Living this way causes us to feel overwhelmed as we feel forced to keep ticking off everything on our to-do lists.

Sometimes it's best to press the pause button on life.

By slowing down, we can reassess our values and set our focus to what is really important in life.

Life is not a race!

The life of Maddy

Let us look at life through Maddy's eyes.

Maddy works as a financial advisor, with a 'typical' Monday to Friday, 40-hour work week. She works eight-hour days. Eight further hours are allocated for sleeping. On her workdays, she spends about five hours on daily tasks that get her by in life, including eating, house chores and commuting to work. This means Maddy has three hours left in the day for herself. We'll call this remaining time, 'you time'.

Let's go further with this. Maddy's yearly schedule would look like this:

- 48 working weeks
- 48 weekends
- Four holiday weeks in a normal year

Calculations

- Spare time of 3 hours x 5 days x 48 working weeks = 720 hours of spare weekday time per year
- 32 weekend hours (16 out of 48 hours goes towards sleep) x 48 weekends = 1,536 weekend hours per year
- Four holiday weeks a year (excluding 224 sleep hours) = 448 holiday hours per year

Total hours of spare time per year = 2,704 hours of 'you time' (720 +1,536 + 448) out of approximately 8,760 total hours (24 hours x 365 days).

Let's say Maddy works until the age of 65. Maddy is 25 years old. That means she has 108,160 available 'you time' hours out of approximately 350,400 total hours (assuming there are 8,760 hours per year).

If we were to apply this to different ages:

- a 30-year-old has 94,640 available hours out of approximately 306,600 total hours left
- a 40-year-old has 67,600 available hours out of approximately 219,000 total hours left
- a 50-year-old has 40,560 available hours out of approximately 131,400 total hours left.

Based on this analysis, Maddy has around 30% of her total time on this planet to do things she wants to do.

This may be an alarming figure for some people, but what is great about this life is you have the ability to change how much 'you time' there is to use.

How would you use this extra time? Would you start a new business? Catch up with friends? Pursue a hobby?

This is why it is recommended we press the pause button or step away from our day-to-day lives.

Give some serious consideration to how you are spending your time because you do not want to get to a time in your life where you regret the opportunities or the risks you did not end up taking.

Treat yourself once in a while, you deserve it

Self-compassion is rare for a lot of people. Our lives can be so chaotic that we do not give ourselves the time to slow down and analyse how we feel.

Are you nervous for an upcoming event? Stressed from work? Ashamed of your past?

We can also push ourselves too far. As discussed earlier in the book, we want to be the best versions of ourselves. This way of life usually results in loss of sleep and raised levels in stress. This is no way for anyone to live.

It is hard to be aware of this unease at the time, but we need to know when it's time to show compassion towards ourselves. Treat yourself once in a while!

If you managed to do a solid week's work, treat yourself to your favourite junk food or a couple of drinks if you want to. Look to spend your down time with loved ones to talk out any stresses and just have a bit of a laugh. Doing this can definitely help put anxieties into perspective.

If your life is getting so stressful you are affected in more ways than one, take a day off, a week off, a month off. Not just from work, but from life.

Of course, our circumstances in life means not all of us can do this but try to have a conversation with the important people in your life — your spouse, your boss, your friends and your family. Let them know you need to step back for a bit and discuss ways you can recharge your batteries. For some people, the longer you take off the better. However, it may be wise to take a different, more sustainable long-term approach, such as only working four days a week. This time off may help you find out what it is you really want to do.

Working ourselves into the ground is no way to live.

We all need a period of time where we can eat what we want, do what we want and do it with the people we want to be around.

Work and money are not as important as we think

A lot of young people have fixed in their head that the expected life goes as follows: work hard in school, get a university degree or trade, get a respectable 9-to-5 job, find someone to have a family with, live happily ever after.

Is this what you really want to do with your life?

It is totally fine if this is how you want to live your life but there are so many more possibilities when it comes to earning a reasonable wage and living a comfortable life.

Many people find it nearly impossible to find a job when they finish their further studies (e.g., uni). Most jobs require experience, but how are you supposed to get a job without experience, right?

Maybe it's wise to wait. Before applying for jobs, try working part-time at the local supermarket, save up and travel for a bit. The options are endless.

The same applies to people who have no idea what they want to do with their adult life. If this is you — there is no rush. Test the waters out and slowly find something you are interested in.

Working all the time is not a way to live. We do not want a lifestyle where we come home and all we have to talk about is work. Let's not put our mates through the torture of having to listen about our work dramas and who is getting promoted over you. If you are unhappy at work, talk to your boss about it or leave.

Money is obviously very influential in the way we live. We need to buy food, pay rent, pay for books and supplies. It is great to work for money to cover essential expenses, however, it is dangerous when we start wanting money to pay for extravagant materialistic things. This makes us crave more, and the luxury items never seem to satisfy us.

This is a similar concept to dopamine-hunting mentioned earlier.

Spend more time focusing on what you love and start buying and working within your means. If you are struggling to get by while travelling the world, pick up a job at a bar for a while.

Do not immerse yourself in work. Spend less time focusing on the outside world and what everyone expects you to do or be. Focus on what you can control and the money will take care of itself. All our paths are different.

Jump back on the horse

- ☹ You slept in and missed your run.
- ☹ You ate junk food when you are supposed to be on a diet.
- ☹ You didn't have time to do your meditation today.
- ☹ You didn't stick to your plan today.
- ☹ You didn't work on your school or uni assignment today.
- ☹ You lost your cool in a stressful moment.
- ☹ You didn't feel like going out to dinner with your mates.
- ☹ You didn't get around to finishing off the DIY deck in the backyard.
- ☹ You forgot to text a friend who you haven't spoken to in a while.
- ☹ You had a drink when you were supposed to be doing Dry July.

Don't be too hard on yourself!

It is awfully difficult to stick to new habits that you try to put in place. It takes time to implement a habit you can stick to and that comfortably fits in to your daily life. Falling off the horse occasionally is just a part of the process.

When you fail to achieve your habit for the day, try to understand why this happened. Was it due to laziness, motivation or fear? When you have established a reason, try to think back to why you are trying to implement this habit into your day-to-day life. You may need to mentally go back to a place where you were at a low point in your life to remember why you want to change. This will hopefully give you a bit of motivation to do better tomorrow.

It also helps to write your new habit on a daily checklist and put it up in a place where you cannot avoid it, for example, the wall next to your bed. The more you see this habit on your checklist, the more motivated you will be to tick it off as soon as possible so you can avoid seeing it for the rest of the day.

Maybe you are being too strict with your new routine. If this is the case, look to give yourself a day or two off to allow your body and mind to relax. Then revisit your goal to see if it might need modifying — at least in the short term.

No matter what it was you did not get around to doing today, remember you are human, and you are not perfect. When you fall off the horse, don't sit in your own guilt or talk down to yourself. Look to rediscover that motivation, remain present and think, *What can I do now that will help me get back on track?* Be positive and look to be a better version of you tomorrow.

Clean your room

Calming

Let's make a to-do list

Everyday make your bed

Accomplishment

No more than five minutes a day to maintain

You will thank yourself

Own up to your mess

Uncompromising attitude to unnecessary belongings

Remove clutter from your benches and floors

Rest in a clean bed

Organised room

Organised mind

Maybe a good idea to empty that bin once in a while

Clean your room is inspired by Jordan Peterson.

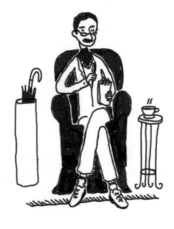

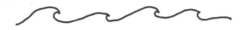

QUOTES & STORIES

WHAT DO OTHER PEOPLE THINK?

'Note that this journey is uniquely yours, no one else's.
So the path has to be your own. You cannot imitate
somebody else's journey and still be true to yourself. Are
you prepared to honor your uniqueness in this way?'

JON KABAT-ZINN, *Wherever You Go, There You Are:
Mindfulness Meditation In Everyday Life*

'Work/life integration seems to me a better goal
than balance. Balance suggests that our lives are
in two parts. The more mindful we are, the less we
compartmentalize our lives.'

ELLEN J. LANGER, *Mindfulness*

'If you are interested in something, you will focus on it,
and if you focus attention on anything, it is likely that
you will become interested in it. Many of the things we
find interesting are not so by nature, but because we
took the trouble of paying attention to them.'

MIHALY CSIKSZENTMIHALYI, *Finding Flow: The Psychology
of Engagement With Everyday Life*

'And I feel like I haven't been making the best choices. There's a lot of things in my life that I need to work on, and sometimes I think that surfing's an indicator, that there's a spiritual message you can get from the things that you do. The results haven't come, and when you're clear-headed and decisive things just seem to fall into place. You've got to get your head right. In everything in life.'

KELLY SLATER, as quoted by Ali Klinkenberg in *Stab Magazine*

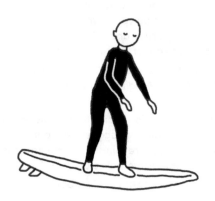

MEDITATION AND
BREATHING

Meditation

Life can often get us down. Maybe you were unfortunate enough to watch an episode of The Masked Singer (seriously, who is watching and why is it still on the air? Couldn't they just stick with the Voice or X Factor? Some TV networks need to...).

Ok ok ok enough ranting, back to the book. Where was I?

Meditation is a great tool to use to bring presence and perspective to your life.

What is it?

An ancient exercise used by many to train the awareness muscle and ultimately relax the mind and body. Many people, including the late Kobe Bryant, surfer Sally Fitzgibbons, Red Hot Chili Peppers frontman Anthony Kiedis and AFL footballer Nat Fyfe have adopted meditation to get themselves in the right frame of mind to perform at a high level.

Do I need to be religious or spiritual to feel the effects of meditation?

No, anyone can do it. You just need to be open-minded.

Is there just one type?

There are literally hundreds of techniques out there. Let's just talk about some that you may have heard of and what they are understood to be:

Guided

Many people start out using guided meditation apps, such as Headspace, or YouTube videos in which an experienced teacher takes you through a simple meditation process. They will tell you when to breathe and what to focus your attention on.

Guided meditations can incorporate many approaches, including the more traditional methods (mentioned below). You can also find specific guided meditations intended for certain people or situations. For example, there are guided meditations designed for sportspeople to complement their training, and others to help students access the right mindset to focus on learning.

Zen

Zen is the Japanese term for meditation. The process involves the meditator holding a comfortable posture, such as a half lotus, while observing the breath. While following the breath in and out of the belly, you let thoughts come and go without judging them or getting wrapped up in them.

It is believed the practice originated from a historical Indian Buddha and has since thrived in countries such as Japan and China. It has grown in popularity in the Western world due to the belief that the practice helps address core issues and questions in people's lives. Awareness is raised and attention is shifted to better understand these problem areas.

Transcendental Meditation (TM)

Originating from teacher, Maharishi Mahesh Yogi, the practice involves sitting in silence and repeating a mantra — a chosen word, phrase or sound — in your mind. If you get lost in thought, you return to the mantra, thus allowing your mind to naturally travel to a less active state.

This technique is used by comedy icon, Jerry Seinfeld. Laugh out loud, more like laugh in silence, am I right? (Sorry, Dad joke).

Chakra

The technique focuses on unlocking and rebalancing the body's core focal points, known as chakras. According to Hindu tradition, there are seven chakras in the human body, including the third eye. However, Buddhists believe there are only four. Check out chakra expert, Anodea

Judith, who has a website and multiple YouTube videos on the topic.

Which one should I use?

Even though there are multiple meditation techniques, a lot of them have similar characteristics including fostering a sense of presence and raising your level of awareness. It is worth doing some more research and experimenting to find the method that best suits you.

CHECK OUT

Anodea Judith, *Eastern Body, Western Mind: Psychology and the Chakra System As a Path to the Self.*

Anodea Judith's website, anodeajudith.com

Jack Kornfield, *Meditation for Beginners.*

Mindworks, 'What is Zen meditation? Benefits & techniques' (web article)

Shunryū Suzuki, *Zen Mind, Beginner's Mind: Informal Talks on Zen Meditation and Practice.*

Theosophical Webinars, 'Anodea Judith — Understanding your chakras' (YouTube video)

Thích Nhat Hanh, *The Miracle of Mindfulness: An Introduction to the Practice of Meditation.*

Meditation at home

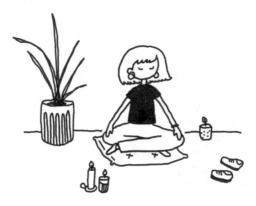

At home, or in a quiet room, is the ideal environment to meditate. This will allow you to focus on the practice without being distracted.

If you choose not to use guided meditation, here is a quick rundown of one common meditation exercise:

1. Sit or lie down in a comfortable position. (Use a pillow if your back gets sore.)

2. Take five deep breaths in and out, focusing on each inhale and exhale as it passes in and out of your mouth.

3. Do a body scan starting from the top of the head down to your toes, bring awareness to each body part. Notice anything that is going on in these body parts — are they warm, cold, tingling?

4. Bring your awareness back to the room and your surroundings, including the chair you may be sitting on.

5. Gently open your eyes.

How do you feel? Calm? Happy? Sad? Confused?

Meditation works differently for each person. Some people are able to focus on the breath for the entire practice, others are thinking about their checklist for the day or what they are going to get for lunch. If that happens for you, simply acknowledge the thought and do your best to return your focus to your breath, mantra or other point of focus for the meditation.

No matter how meditation goes for you each time, keep persisting. You may not feel the effects of meditation immediately but try to use the practice over a few months. If you use meditation within your day-to-day life for an extended period of time, you will find your outlook on life and your mental state both change.

As you continue this practice, the little things will not get to you as much. Getting stuck in traffic will be seen as an opportunity to take in what is around you — the vibrant colours of nature, a cute dog on a walk, or the cool breeze on your face if you open a window.

Using meditation, the paths we take towards a present and happy lifestyle often come with our own personal challenges. If you want to persist with meditation but need some help, there are plenty of personal or group sessions you can attend where a meditation expert can give you some tips on how to meditate effectively.

Meditation everywhere

'When the mind is allowed to relax,
inspiration often follows.'
PHIL JACKSON, *Eleven Rings: The Soul of Success*

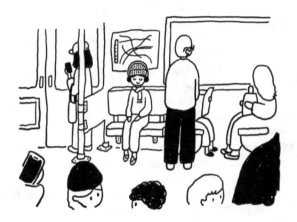

Meditation at home is not always possible. You may have a very busy morning where you need to make sure everyone is taken care of and various tasks are completed before you go to work. If you are really not a morning person and value your sleep too much to wake up early, try meditating away from home.

I know what you're thinking and no I don't want you to get into a meditation pose in the middle of a meeting. Rather, the practice asks you to do the following:

1. Wherever you are, be more aware of your surroundings. Pay attention to the smaller things. What colour is the window frame? How does your hand feel on the table? Are there any unusual noises around the room?

2. Pay attention to your breath.

3. Notice your thoughts, without judgement.

If you have a long commute to work on the train, you can put your headphones in, close your eyes and follow a guided meditation. If you are concerned about looking weird, do not worry! It will look like you are simply having a little nap, which is extremely common on public transport. Then, when you are walking from the train station to the office, notice the air, trees and people around you. This will force your mind to focus on something apart from yourself and any negative thoughts you may be dealing with.

Some people will stand in the shower and think about what they have to do that day, or about something they wished they said. Shower time is the perfect opportunity to workout your mindfulness and awareness muscles. Feel the water vibrating on your head, notice the little water bubbles on the shower screen, be aware of how the shower experience makes you feel as a whole. Is it making you feel warm? Cold? Relaxed? Tense?

Use meditation when you are at work, watching a netball game, walking the dog, kicking the footy, or even when you are watching Netflix. The more you meditate, the quicker it will become a habit. You are not going to be 'Zen' 24/7, but you will be able to prevent yourself being caught up in your own emotions and thoughts.

CHECK OUT

Jon Kabat-Zinn, *Wherever You Go, There You Are: Mindfulness Meditation in Everyday Life.*

Breathing is not just something that keeps us alive

'Breathing in, I calm body and mind. Breathing out, I smile. Dwelling in the present moment I know this is the only moment.'

THICH NHAT HANH, *Being Peace*

It is odd how little attention we pay to our breathing. The body's breathing operates on autopilot for most of the day and we completely take this for granted. Life would be very different if we took the same approach to eating, chatting with a mate or pursuing a hobby.

We've all had this experience: you're stressed and trying to let your anger out and someone comes up to you and says, 'Mate calm down, take a breath.' For a lot of people, this just makes things worse. Why? It seems completely crazy to think people prefer being mad over being calm.

As much as we hate hearing this, focusing on our breath actually works. It is not just the breath that is calming us down, but also the awareness of our body and emotions.

When we become more aware of these things, we are able to look at our feelings through a different scope. Rather than being something that can hurt us, we allow ourselves to see these emotions merely as thoughts. Nothing more, nothing less.

We discussed the body scan earlier. In this practice, we are able to 'breathe into' particular areas of our bodies. Take a moment to breathe and notice how your belly rises on the inhale and becomes smaller on the exhale. This exercise helps us relax our mind and body as we are focusing our attention on the breath and not on the thoughts challenging us.

You can take this practice almost anywhere — maybe don't try it underwater though.

Never take your breath for granted. Not only is it an avenue for a calmer mind, body and spirit but more importantly, it is keeping you alive.

CHECK OUT

Dr Kasim Al-Mashat, 'How mindfulness meditation redefines pain, happiness & satisfaction' https://www.youtube.com/watch?v=JVw LjC5etEQ

QUOTES & STORIES

WHAT DO OTHER PEOPLE THINK?

PHIL JACKSON

'When the mind is allowed to relax, inspiration often follows.' — *Eleven Rings: The Soul of Success*

KOBE BRYANT

Kobe was one of the hardest working athletes to ever live. As he got older, he learned to work smarter and not harder. In a video on the YouTube channel, Thrive Global, Kobe said he did about fifteen minutes of meditation a day. He said he would meditate in the morning, as he thought the practice 'sets me up for the rest of the day'. In the video, Kobe set an assignment for newcomers to meditation:

1. Get an additional 30 minutes of sleep.
2. Start with just five minutes of meditation each day.

SALLY FITZGIBBONS

In an interview with Body and Soul, Sally calls regular meditation non-negotiable. 'When I first open my eyes, I pay attention to being centred and focusing my breath through a meditation practice,' she says. 'Just committing to 10 minutes a day, where I have a single focus, can go a long way. [It helps me] go about my day calmly, connect to what I'm doing instead of rushing all the way to the end of the day without a conscious breath'.

ANTHONY KIEDIS

In an interview with Rolling Stone, the Red Hot Chili Peppers frontman discusses his pre-show routine: 'You can't go from zero to 100 miles per hour without preparing,' he says. While bandmate, Flea, 'gets gig-ready by playing for an hour and then running around the arena' according to the article's author, Kory Grow, Kiedis' own habits are a little different: 'I meditate, I pray ... I'm pretty intense about it,' he says. 'I think the best way to perform is to be relaxed ... I want to be excited to play.'

NAT FYFE

Nat was initially sceptical about the benefits of meditation, according to Michael Dulaney of the ABC's Mindfully, but he discovered that 'preparing for the mental side of the game was as important as the physical side'. He now takes anywhere from five minutes to 35 minutes throughout the day to meditate and raise his awareness. 'Most mornings, I'll start with some sort of ritual, whether it's going to the beach or sitting in front of my fire, or something that just quickly realigns me and welcomes me into the day,' Fyfe said. 'But most of my meditation I find I do at night ... I sit in a quiet place in my room or my hotel or wherever I am around the country, and I'll listen to focus on my breathing and stillness.' Fyfe added the principles extend well beyond the sporting field. 'I think to catch yourself through everyday life, whether things are going good or badly, and just intervene with a bit of meditation or stillness ... the more effectively you're going to function as a human.'

FORGETTING
THE PAST,
NOT OVERTHINKING
THE FUTURE
AND BEING IN
THE PRESENT

Shame and guilt from your past

Shame and guilt are dark feelings that can force us to think we are not worthy or lovable. We can often experience these feelings as a result of traumatic events from our past.

We all have things we regret doing in life: 'I wish I never teased that kid at school'; 'I wish I spent more time with my mum and dad'; 'I should have taken that promotion'.

You are not defined by the things you have done in your past.

Be forgiving about what you have done and understand it was impossible for you to know all the answers in every stage of your life. Use the lessons from your mistakes to grow and become a better person.

For those of us who are holding on to shame, we may feel like other people could use our past to attack, exploit or humiliate us. It is important to know, unless you are a well-known celebrity, any shame you are holding on to will most likely never be known by the majority of the population—there are over 7.5 billion people on the planet for crying out loud.

If we keep our deepest, darkest shames hidden, they will eat away at us. These shameful thoughts are unlikely to be as bad as we may think, and we too often catastrophise what would happen if people found out about who we truly are.

As shame researcher Brené Brown shares in her book, *Daring Greatly: How the Courage to Be Vulnerable Transforms the Way We Live, Love, Parent, and Lead*:

> If we can share our story with someone who responds with empathy and understanding, shame can't survive ... Numb the dark and you numb the light.

It is so important to open up when we can. Look to a friend, a family member, a psychologist or councillor to allow these dark thoughts to come into the light. A lot of our thoughts are relatable to other people's experiences and speaking of our shame to others can show us how truly accepting and loving people can be when we are vulnerable.

Opening up can be one of the most scary and uncomfortable experiences a person has to go through, but it is a massive step towards keeping shame and guilt away from our day-to-day lives.

Please refer to the chapter 'Trauma, shame and embarrassment' for more on a similar topic.

CHECK OUT

Brené Brown, *Daring Greatly: How the Courage to Be Vulnerable Transforms the Way We Live, Love, Parent, and Lead.*

The most important moment is right now: taking small steps towards your big goals

'The past has no power over the present moment.'

ECKHART TOLLE, *The Power of Now*

One of the most difficult parts about remaining present is stopping our thoughts from taking over. This is more difficult to do in places or situations where we experience high levels of stress. It is important to realise that when we are aware of our thoughts, especially when we feel trapped in thought or emotion, we have the power to take our focus away from this mindset and focus on the here and now.

The mind loves to focus on scenarios that have either already happened or are about to happen. We need to remember these scenarios are not real; they are not standing right in front of you.

Your brain can form mental images based on your experiences, but they are NOT REAL. The only thing that is REAL is what is staring you right in the face. The here. The now.

If you have a major assignment due in two weeks, it is not going to get done if you are sitting with thoughts of fear or guilt about the assignment. You can control what you do today! Doing a little bit now is going to get your momentum going, and the lessons you learn along the way will allow you to complete the assignment with a largely reduced amount of stress. A great place to start is by ranking the parts of the assignment from easiest to hardest. Begin on the easiest part first and work your way up.

The more time we are stuck in thought, the less time we have to be productive and intentional. Begin to catch yourself when your mind is stuck in negative or unnecessary thoughts. Start looking at your life now – not yesterday and not tomorrow. Your life is today.

CHECK OUT

Eckhart Tolle, *The Power of Now: A Guide to Spiritual Enlightenment.*

Catch yourself when you are not present

No one has gone through life completely unfazed. We all go through our own rollercoaster ride, encountering many frustrations along the way.

A common example is getting stuck in traffic. The immediate response to this is anger and impatience as you want to get from point A to point B as soon as possible. Negative thoughts rush through your head: 'I should be there by now!' or 'If only this dickhead would move over to the left lane'. However, if you were to stop and pay attention to your emotions and thoughts in the situation, your mindset would soon change. Do not judge these thoughts or label them in anyway, just notice them like passing cars on a road – if you'll excuse me for stretching the metaphor.

It is key to realise when these thoughts are taking over our behaviour. When you feel overwhelmed, disconnect yourself from the situation and from any negative thoughts you may be having. Try to pay attention to the present. When we catch ourselves in this pattern, we begin to feel a lot more relaxed as we rationalise the situation in a much calmer manner.

We can catch ourselves out anywhere, such as:

- during a confrontation with friends
- in a boring work meeting
- before making a speech in front of our class.

We are surrounded by things that constantly stimulate us — advertising, social media, noise pollution — making it easier to become stressed. Worse, we often become so accustomed to these many competing messages fighting for our attention, we end up giving in to them while trying to relax. How often do you reach for your phone to scroll through Facebook or Insta when you have a few minutes of peace?

Mindfulness is reached when you begin to be present all the time. This takes constant realisation of moments when you are deep in thought about the past and future, or even a moment that's occurring in the now. Consistently realising you are not present is a key factor to mindfulness.

Future thinking is good, but do not obsess

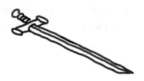

Game of Thrones spoiler alert below. I repeat, Game of Thrones spoiler alert.

Most of us have bucket lists we want to tick off before we die. Even making New Year's resolutions can fool us into thinking these achievements will be the ones to unlock our happiness.

We may say things like: 'Once I get that job, everything will be perfect', 'Once I have taken that big trip around the world, then I will be happy', 'When those renovations are done, life will be easier'.

It can be difficult not to obsess about what is going to happen in the future. We plan scenarios in our mind that have not even happened yet.

For example, maybe you agreed to see your boyfriend/ girlfriend's parents this weekend. You have been dreading going all week because you think the parents are going to judge you and think negatively of you.

For times like these, you just need to accept the decision you made — in this instance, to meet the parents. Once you do accept the decision, you also need to accept the fact there may be hiccups when that time comes around, but also learn to realise you will not die from most of the things you worry about.

Happiness is not something we can predict will happen in the future. Happiness can come from acceptance of your current life and knowing you are making positive steps towards being a better person.

We get caught up in ticking things off our list, always working towards some future goal. If we focus too much on the future and not enough on the here and how, this can end up making us feel anxious.

Life is similar to a TV show. The main characters go through ups and downs which build their personalities, attitudes and behaviours. You don't want to skip right to the end.

Let's take Arya Stark from Game of Thrones. She watches her father being executed, escapes Kings Landing and has to fend for herself at around eleven years old. She gets knocked out by the Hound while trying to save her family from the red wedding, befriends him and then has to leave him dying under a tree, and forfeits her identity to join the Faceless Men. These are just a few of the obstacles Arya had to face before becoming the hero of the show, killing the Night King and, as a result, saving so many lives.

This is why it is important to be focused on the journey and not the end result. Looking too far ahead forces you to lose sight of the work and dedication needed to reach that end goal. Be as present as you can and focus on what you can control today. The rest will take care of itself.

Whatever will be, will be

We get stuck in the mud from time to time, especially when we are preoccupied with thoughts about things that are completely out of our control. The more we get ourselves into this position, the more anxious, depressed and stressed we are likely to feel. We need to shift our attention from thinking about all our long-term fears and anxieties and try to pay more attention to what we can influence and control today.

Focus on what we can control

It is difficult to get a grasp on what exactly is in the realm of our control, especially when we have thoughts constantly running through our head and we're filled with self-doubt and anxiety. That's why it is important to shift our attention.

We are able to control many facets of our lives including how much sleep we get, who we hang out with and what job we work in. Why not control how we focus our attention?

A way to focus on what we can control is to shift our attention to anything that is real and in front of us. For example, when going for a run, we focus on 'left foot, right foot' or when tuning into an audiobook, we invest ourselves in everything being read.

Pursue a hobby you enjoy. You can find meditational qualities in many hobbies, including:

- Painting — making art really helps us express ourselves in the way we would like, bringing any emotions we have inside out onto a plain canvas

- Surfing — the waves, the calming sound of the ocean, the shift in attention to trying to better yourself each time you try to catch a wave

- Learning an instrument — similar to painting, expressing yourself through music can be a great way to stimulate positive thoughts or relax.

Letting go

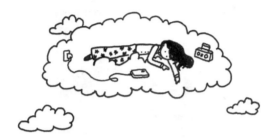

It is easy to become overwhelmed by our racing minds. We do not want to ignore our mental commentary; we want to acknowledge it is happening. We want to make sure we are not avoiding our thoughts and trying to sweep them under the rug; they are not going to go away.

We need to learn to 'let go' and let thoughts happen in their own organic way.

When we start letting go, it is almost like floating on air as though there is nothing weighing us down. This is because we have stopped obsessing over parts of our life that do not encourage growth. We begin to stop worrying about things like a slightly crooked nose, that time we tripped over on stage or how smart we sound in a social setting.

In order to let go, we also need to learn to forgive ourselves. We should all cut ourselves some slack and be kind to ourselves. When we start to feel worried about the future or memories from the past, we should try to remember how good we are as a person and be grateful for what we are in this moment.

By reading this book, you are making the right decision because you are trying to improve yourself. Good job you!

Something that is really helpful to a lot of people is getting off your phone. We talk about this more in the chapter, *Stop dopamine hunting*.

Mortality

'The fear of death follows from the fear of life. A man who lives fully is prepared to die at any time.'

COMMONLY ATTRIBUTED TO MARK TWAIN

When a new life is brought into the world, it is seen as one of the most beautiful moments humans can experience. The whole process is beautiful, from the decision to start a family to the excitement that builds during the pregnancy period, and finally the day when the baby is here in the world for everyone to hold and love. This cute little baby will get to grow up to experience an amazing world filled with hopes and opportunities.

However, when death comes around, it is often met with great sadness, regret, anger and a lot of tears. Those close to the person will never get to see this person they loved ever again.

What is most important is how you perceive death.

Death of a loved one can be an awful experience, but we can learn to accept death in a more mindful way. Yes, pain for the loss will still be felt but by approaching death more mindfully we can find it a little easier to make peace with death. This is best achieved through living a life that is mindful. This way, we are better equipped to deal with these experiences while being able to appreciate how fragile and meaningful life is.

It's a reality a lot of people do not want to face — we are all going to die.

Not being aware of your mortality will most likely lead you through a life that is unfulfilling. This may include being stuck in a job you hate, hanging around with people who stress you out or getting smashed every weekend at the same bar. Living in this way will more than likely lead you to wake up in twenty years and think,

'Where did that time go?'

People can also be attracted to drugs and alcohol to escape their fears of death and the shitty life they have to live. This is a short-term fix that will only lead to further fears of death.

As touched on a little earlier, being mindful of death and your own mortality is vital for understanding how precious life is. An effective way of becoming more mindful with regards to death is to accept it. Knowing your days are numbered and treating every moment with complete care will lead you to a much more fulfilling life. This may mean you have to reconsider your current life, including your job, where you live, social life, diet and hobbies. This will mean a lot more risk-taking to change your life. However, as long as you are making changes for the right reasons, there are far more risks if you don't.

Make sure you wake up in twenty years with an optimistic look on life. Look forward to what is to come and celebrate what you have done to get yourself into that position. Start today. Live a life where you only take actions that you will be proud of in twenty years.

CHECK OUT

Héctor García and Francesc Miralles, *Ikigai: The Japanese Secret to a Long and Happy Life*.

Headspace, 'Mindful death' (web article).

Caitlin Doughty, 'It's never too early to start thinking about your own death', Vox (web article).

Diary writing

Diary writing, or journalling, is one of the key contributors to connecting our state of happiness and mindfulness.

Writing down our thoughts forces our anxieties, fears and stresses, relating to both the past and future, to lose their edge. By transferring all of this to paper, it shines light on our dark thoughts. It is then a lot easier for us to let go of the negative thoughts.

The process also helps us to perceive our thoughts and manage our emotions. We increase self-awareness as we can now see our thoughts in third person. It is almost as if we are reading someone else's story and are able to learn from their experiences. We start understanding and relating to the environment we live in more every day.

We may also see certain patterns in our thought process and behaviour. Realising these patterns exist can help us prioritise our problems and focus on areas of our lives that need the most attention.

A lot of people tend to use diary writing as a chance to write down things they are grateful for. Doing this increases self-awareness and helps us focus on the good rather than the bad in our lives.

Try to write in a diary every day for a month. Dedicate a regular time every day and write about anything that is on your mind or that has happened during that day. It does not matter how significant or small the events or thoughts are. Try to write at least two pages in a small booklet or journal. Once you have written your thoughts, jot down three things you are grateful for. Think of this experience in the same way as doing daily exercise. If you miss a day, it's okay! Get back on the horse tomorrow.

Write anything — it's your diary. For example:

- *I am sick of Jack being such a fuckwit at work ... (half a page)*
- *Why hasn't Jen texted me back still? ... (full page)*
- *I have to take my dog to the vet this weekend, I hope everything is alright ... (half a page)*

Three things I am grateful for:

- *Having a family I can always rely on to offer me support and advice when I need it*
- *Having a stable job and income that can buy me the essentials I need and some luxuries on top of that*
- *Being able to come home to my dog who loves me whether I had a good day or a bad day at work.*

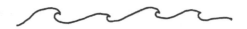

QUOTES & STORIES

WHAT DO OTHER PEOPLE THINK?

'If we open a quarrel between the past and the present
we shall find that we have lost the future.'

WINSTON CHURCHILL, 'Their Finest Hour'

'Patience is a form of wisdom. It demonstrates that we
understand and accept the fact that sometimes things
must unfold in their own time.'

JON KABAT-ZINN, *Full Catastrophe Living: Using the
Wisdom of Your Body and Mind to Face Stress, Pain,
and Illness*

'Realize deeply that the present moment is all you have.
Make the NOW the primary focus of your life.'

ECKHART TOLLE, *The Power of Now: A Guide To Spiritual
Enlightenment*

'We cannot selectively numb emotions, when we
numb the painful emotions, we also numb the positive
emotions.'

BRENÉ BROWN, *The Gifts Of Imperfection*

'There's no such thing as a minor lapse of awareness. You're either present with what is — right here, right now — or you're someplace else.'

GAY HENDRICKS, *The First Rule Of Ten*

'Mindfulness can encourage creativity when the focus is on the process and not the product.'

ELLEN J. LANGER, *Mindfulness*

"Only we humans worry about the future, regret the past, and blame ourselves for the present."

RICK HANSON, *Buddha's Brain: The Practical Neuroscience of Happiness, Love, and Wisdom*

STOP DOPAMINE
HUNTING

What is dopamine?

Dopamine is a neurotransmitter produced by nerve cells in the brain. It acts as a messenger between neurons, and works with other neurotransmitters and hormones, such as serotonin and adrenaline. Dopamine is often released when you achieve something the brain considers to be rewarding or pleasurable. Sugary foods, going for a run and sex are just a few things that can stimulate the body to release dopamine.

Dopamine plays a big role in shaping a person's behaviour. It can be a great way to improve focus on learning and sticking to a task. It is also a great helper in boosting motivation to actually get up and do that task.

It is important to note that we need to be cautious of things that can cause a significant spike in dopamine. Drugs and alcohol are known to make people feel on top of the world, but when that dopamine high wears off, people usually feel down in the dumps.

If dopamine levels are low, this can often lead to a negative effect on your mental health.

Schizophrenia and Attention Deficit Hyperactivity Disorder (ADHD) are common disorders relating to too much or too little dopamine in the brain.

A healthy lifestyle and meditation are just a couple of ways of boosting your dopamine in a sustainable way. They can also help us to become more aware when dopamine is starting to take over, for example when you start craving that large pizza.

The way dopamine works, and the brain as a whole, is truly remarkable. We should be grateful for this messenger system the brain has put together because if we did not have it, we would never feel excited for a date, or experience euphoria after achieving a long-term goal.

I hope that, at some point, this book will give you a little boost in dopamine along the way.

CHECK OUT

Health Direct, 'Dopamine', (web article).

Ann Pietrangelo, 'How does dopamine affect the body?' in Healthline (web article).

Smitha Bhandari (editor), 'What is Dopamine?' in WebMD (web article).

The internet can be helpful, but use it carefully

How do we expect to ever stay focused when there is a giant, giant, GIANT world where we can find and learn about anything, from diagnosing the rash you have on your arm to finding a recipe for a traditional banana bread?

With so much to see and do on the internet, it often leads to us becoming distracted from the initial purpose of jumping on our computer, phone or tablet in the first place.

Have you ever noticed how many times you go back to all of your saved 'watch later' videos? How many webpages or tabs have you bookmarked to visit another time? How you're still getting notifications from a Facebook group that you liked back in high school? A lot of people never go back to these things, because they are always seeking new information.

The situation today is definitely a lot more advanced compared to thirty years ago where the best place to find information was the library. Nowadays, we are flooded with apps giving us notifications on the latest stock prices, injury news from your favourite sport, and foreign political news.

We don't even have to try to learn anymore. All the information we need — and a lot that we don't — is right at our fingertips.

How can we manage this so we don't get caught up in a never-ending cycle, clicking from one video or site to another?

Notice when you are not sticking to the intended task. When you do realise you are off track, close or save the window you were on and come back to it when you have finished.

Similarly, try not to multitask. Look to tick off the tasks you want to complete on the internet, one thing at a time. A good way to do this is setting a daily time limit for your internet use.

When you feel overwhelmed from information overload, close your device and go for a walk. Nothing beats getting some fresh air!

Alcohol, smoking, drugs, caffeine

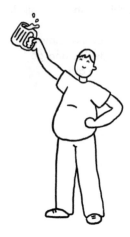

We have the option of indulging in all sorts of stimulants these days. Some are used to relax us; others are used to keep us awake and others are used to give us more confidence in social situations.

Alcohol

> *'To alcohol! The cause of — and solution to — all of life's problems.'*
>
> HOMER SIMPSON, *The Simpsons* (S8 E18)

Binge drinking has become a large part of Australian culture. A young Aussie may spend their Saturday night in this way:

- Go to a mate's house for pre-drinks.
- Get through as much of your ten-pack as humanly possible before heading out to a festival or a night on the town.

- Spend a lot of your time in queues, hitting the D-floor, talking to strangers who you will never see again and shouting your mates (and sometimes strangers) $15 drinks left, right and centre. (Don't forget SHOTS!)
- After Daryl Braithwaite's *Horses* is played at the end of the night for the 167th week in a row, it is probably time to call it a night.
- Get drive-through at Macca's on the Uber-ride home.
- Pass out after your second nugget.
- Wake up the next morning — hopefully in your own bed.

We are stopping here because it is obviously the start of the next day but also because we want you to think of the feeling you wake up with the next day, and the days following after a 'big one'. Anxiety? Shame? Embarrassment? Sad? Angry?

However you may be feeling, it will most likely be not so great.

Most of us would pin this down to the alcohol being the reason for feeling so terrible, however, it is important to also factor in a lack of sleep, dehydration and a poor diet.

According to Queensland Health, as your body is working to get alcohol out of your system, blood sugar levels drop, which can stress the brain out. This can lead to increased feelings of anxiety.

We use alcohol to give us more confidence and help us relax. It is a popular way of escaping from the real world.

We can wake up feeling a lot happier and more relaxed if we decide to take a more mindful approach to our drinking.

THIS DOES NOT NECESSARILY MEAN GIVING UP DRINKING.

For the binge drinker I described earlier, there are some alternatives you can choose to implement:

1. Incorporate water rounds with your drinking. Get a glass of water after every drink or two to keep you more switched on and a lot more hydrated. Use apps, such as Hydro Coach, to send you reminders to drink water.

2. Start early, finish early. Make it clear you have to be home earlier. Make sure your excuse, or lie, is believable and consistent. You will be appreciated by your mates for making the effort to get there earlier. Even better, make an actual commitment for the morning after. Your sleeping pattern will thank you.

3. Extend the time between drinks. This means drinking a lot more slowly than your mates. You can implement this strategy by setting a timer or keeping a conscious eye on the clock, making sure you buy a drink when the clock says so.

4. When feeding the late-night food craving, do your best to pick a healthier alternative. Try vegan! A better option would be to wait for the morning after to eat. Food right before bed is pretty bad for your health in its own right.

5. Do not go out with the mentality of drinking to get smashed. Focus on having a controlled, low number of drinks. If you are looking to meet the love of your life while on the piss, they definitely will not want to be near you if you are off your face.

6. If something is bugging you from the night before, journal it. Write everything that happened and how it all made you feel.

7. Take a moment to count your breaths. This will help you become mindful of any alcohol cravings and the environment around you.

Smoking

Australian ads were interesting during the early 2000s. One of the more graphic was the quit smoking series. Perhaps you remember the person on the hospital bed with tubes coming out everywhere, trying to scare all smokers into quitting. This may have worked for some people but not all — quitting is very hard!

Let's be honest. If you smoke, you have a pretty good idea that every drag you take is probably not doing the best for your physical health. What you may not realise is that it is also negatively affecting your mental health. This is largely due to the nicotine.

When a drag of a cigarette is taken, the nicotine sets off a rush of dopamine to the brain, which makes us feel good. This starts a bad behaviour pattern, as each smoke you take is providing a reward to the brain: 'Yes, thank you. Please keep doing this.'

Tools we can use to help our smoking-free or smoking-less journey include:

- Meditation — this allows us to step back from our behaviours and desires. Regular practice stops us from acting on emotion or instinct and pushes us towards regulating our bad habits.

- Smoking triggers — identifying these triggers, such as locations, times of day and social settings is essential. As we notice these triggers, we become more aware and can better prepare ourselves to be mindful of any urge.

- Journalling — write down your progress every day. When we do this, we can identify what is working and what is not. This tool also keeps us on track and accountable for our actions.

I am not here to provide you a clear-cut way of nipping this in the bud. The aim is to provide smokers with a different way of thinking about their addiction. As with any medical issue, you should consult your doctor for personalised advice if you are having trouble quitting on your own.

Caffeine

Caffeine is used to kick-start the day for a lot of people. We use it for multiple purposes, including sport, work and even driving a car.

However, it is possible to become overstimulated, leading to difficulty relaxing and focusing. What makes this worse is caffeine is considered to be a highly addictive substance. It can lead us to feel anxious and agitated, and it can increase blood pressure.

Let's go over some ways we can be more mindful when consuming caffeine.

Remember, THIS DOES NOT NECESSARILY MEAN GIVING UP CAFFEINE.

Coffee is very popular among Western civilisations. People can drink three or more cups of coffee a day. If you feel that coffee is having an effect on your mindfulness, look to reducing this. The same can be applied to those who use energy drinks or tea.

Maybe try a day without caffeine. Then two days, and so on. Over time, you may be surprised by how well you can function without your morning cup of coffee. Maybe go for a morning walk instead?

It is also vital to make sure our caffeine intake is not impacting our sleep. Our focus is better when we've come off a full night's sleep, without caffeine, compared to having less than eight hours of sleep and fuelling up on coffee. For this reason, it's best to avoid caffeinated drinks after around 2:00 pm.

If you're feeling experimental, try to live by the saying 'no brew after two' for a month. By repeating this message to yourself, you are further reinforcing your caffeine-reducing habit and also giving your body a greater chance of sleep when it comes to bedtime.

Drugs

'I was a proper smackhead, crackhead, and look at me now! No smack, no crack, still problems, still crazy ... I have freedom now and you can have freedom too.'

RUSSELL BRAND

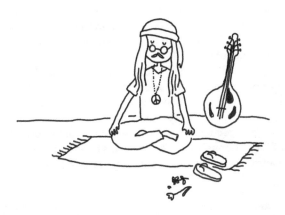

Most of us know UK comedian and actor, Russell Brand.

In his younger years, Russell lived a lifestyle filled with drugs, alcohol, sex and other destructive vices. He became addicted to drugs at very young age. As Russell started to earn more money and drugs became more available, his addiction only got worse.

Russell regarded himself as an instinctive person. This, along with negative personal experiences, including eating disorders and porn addiction in his younger years may have impacted his substance abuse.

After a lot of hard work through personal discovery, rehab and using methods such as the Twelve Steps of Alcoholics Anonymous (AA) and other related recovery programs, Russell started to find his own spiritual awakening. He began to better understand his mind, his emotions and the personal impacts of the world around him.

Now, he regularly uses tools, such as yoga and meditation, to better connect with himself and his emotions. He also puts a lot of his time into helping others who are going through similar experiences.

He has been clean since 2002 and is now one of the most prominent advocates for spirituality and wellbeing. Like all of us, he is still on his spiritual journey and is still learning about his world.

If you take the time to discover yourself and make the effort to understand yourself, you can be mindful of any addictions or cravings you may have for drugs or anything else for that matter.

I highly recommend you check out Russell Brand's YouTube channel or podcasts he has been in, such as his appearance on the *Joe Rogan Experience* podcast.

Overall

The ideal scenario for each of these — alcohol, smoking, caffeine and illicit drugs — would be to go cold turkey and see the effects. However, you need to take into account your current situation and environment, as some people would receive a massive shock to their system if they just dropped a drug they were dependent on. Take small steps, regulate these substances to suit your lifestyle and be sure to live within your means.

If you believe you are facing an addiction issue, please seek professional help. There are plenty of specialists who can provide you with a plan and ongoing support to help get your addiction under control.

CHECK OUT

The Chopra Well, 'Russell Brand's Story — Overcoming Addiction Through Yoga' (YouTube video).

Jess Hardiman, 'Russell Brand is celebrating 15 years free from drugs and alcohol', Lad Bible (web article).

Queensland Health, '10 weird things you might not know alcoholic drinks are doing to your body' (web article)

Hydro Coach (hydrocoach.com) is one of many available apps to help you remind yourself to drink more water.

Rich Roll, 'The awakening of Russell Brand', Rich Roll Podcast (YouTube video).

TMhome.com, 'Russell Brand meditated every day and this is what happened to him' (web article).

Distractions are everywhere

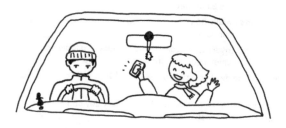

When you drive, you are able to manage multiple distractions while following the road rules.

Judd is driving himself and his best mate Tommo to get some lunch. Tommo loves to have a yarn—a chat for you less ocker readers. He asks for Judd's phone passcode because he wants to chuck some Fisher on the Spotify queue.

'Yeeeee boi!'—Tommo's bangers start blasting out and he is getting right into it, tapping on the dashboard, clapping and just making a downright ruckus.

Two minutes later, Tommo yells, 'Look, look, look! It's Jemma Stone from school.'

Judd quickly turns his head to make sure it is her, and Tommo proceeds to reminisce about her beauty throughout his schooling years. Judd then enters a suburb he has found difficult to drive around in the past, due to tricky intersections and turns.

Tommo receives a phone call from his mate from work and puts him on loudspeaker. They are talking about Tommo's date last night with his new lover.

Judd's stress levels rise. His concentration on these challenging roads is slowly being directed elsewhere.

Scenario 1

Judd thinks about asking Tommo to turn off his loud speaker but decides against it as he is confident in his ability to concentrate with these distractions. He approaches a difficult right turn at an intersection. Judd forgets to give way to oncoming traffic and, as a result, clips the back of another car. No one was hurt in the incident, but Judd had to fork out over a grand in repairs. He copped a grilling from the other driver and felt terrible knowing he could have seriously hurt the driver and his mate.

Scenario 2

Judd asks Tommo politely, 'Mate, can you please just chuck your phone off loudspeaker for a sec?' After Tommo agrees to this, Judd confidently navigates the difficult roads in a calm manner. No one gets hurt.

Making the right choice

This is not supposed to come across like a road safety ad but it does show how dealing with distractions can be key in getting the best results. The key to dealing with distractions is to not lose your cool and be able to recognise when you are being distracted. Understand that whatever is distracting you can usually be managed and regulated. Do whatever you need to do to become more present, whether that is breathing exercises, meditation or something else that works for you. This will allow you to feel much calmer and make rational decisions.

For example:

- Students studying for an exam would turn their phones off.
- Readers would turn off any background noise, such as a radio or TV.

- Golf crowds should be completely silent when Tiger Woods is taking a swing.

Judd was faced with many distractions — music, girls and loud mates. In Scenario 2, Judd was able to manage his distractions and continue the drive. We are very capable of being calm and focused, even when our environment is chaotic.

On the other hand, in times of complete calm, it is possible to get distracted. During meditation, we will often find ourselves lost in thought. People often give up on meditation due to this, saying, 'I can't do this anymore; I just cannot focus enough on the practice.'

In times like this, you need to be kinder and more forgiving of yourself when you do become distracted. Work on noticing when you are not present. You can track of this by keeping note of how many times you were able to shift your attention back to the present moment.

The world we live in today is full of distractions – phones, media, social media, apps and advertisements are just some of the many things that give us hours of (sometimes) pointless pleasure and keeping us away from tasks that are important to us. If we remove these distractions from our day-to-day lives, we allow ourselves the best opportunity to maintain our focus and get the most out of our day.

CHECK OUT

The YouTube channel Better Ideas has a heap of videos on dealing with distractions and being intentional with your time.

Phones and social media — stop scrolling, read a book

For some, lying in bed is often accompanied by having a browse of all the social media apps, checking through all the notifications, stories and posts that can *obviously* not wait until tomorrow. When you put the phone down to go to bed, a notification flashes up on your screen. You pick your phone up and proceed to engage in another 30-minute Snapchat conversation with a friend.

Social media was supposed to bring us closer together. You can connect with long-lost friends, someone you are attracted to at work but are too nervous to approach in person, or family members who live overseas. You can join groups that appeal to your interests, making you feel a sense of belonging and acceptance. Social media is even a great way to sell any junk you do not need. It sounds like a great tool for society, right?

Actually, if we look at the other end of the spectrum, social media has made people feel more alone and isolated than ever before – especially the people closest to us. How many of us get home from work or school and, instead of having the typical 'How was your day?' conversation at the dinner table, scroll through our social media platforms and DM our mates?

Nothing is more precious than communicating with loved ones, face-to-face. As humans, we need to see facial expressions and hear emotion in someone's voice to feel a true connection. We were not designed to send texts and DMs to people we can easily meet with.

Looking through social media for hours on end can lead us to feel really down on ourselves. We often look through the highlight reel of people we envy. We want to be friends with them or live a lifestyle more like theirs. It can also lead to overthinking and build unwarranted rivalries and feuds among friendships groups because posts and pictures can easily be misinterpreted and messages can be said more openly as there is no face-to-face contact.

We need to become more mindful with the ways we use our phones and any social media platforms. This is hard to do when it seems like our whole lives are on these platforms. If you feel like social media is distracting you from your life and is making you less mindful, try these techniques:

- Realise that dopamine hits should be for things that actually contribute to your life and your overall wellbeing. Being aware that dopamine hits from notifications and likes are not contributing to your life will help you to feel less emotion to any alerts from your phone.

- Turn off all notifications. This is great for people who need to focus at work. Your messages and tagged posts can wait until you get home; your friends are not going to abandon you for not seeing their latest beach bod transformation Insta.

- Regularly evaluate your social media accounts to figure out which ones are making you happy or helping you in the 'real' world and deactivate the ones that are not. You will come to realise your world does not revolve around your online presence.

- Filter your feed so you can only see posts or people that actually make you happy. This will mean you can scroll with a lot less worry and stress as you will often find little pieces of wisdom or knowledge that could help you in your real-world life.

- Don't post to make yourself look cool. Post to make yourself happy or to make the world a better place.

- Before you go on your phone, set out your intention. Are you quickly messaging a friend the time to meet for lunch? Are you checking the promo code for tickets to a festival? Whatever your reason is, try your best to stick to that main intention and if you get distracted, calmly realise you are going off track and put your phone down.

- If someone posts something you don't like, try to not take it personally or get frustrated by it. This also applies to a negative comment directed towards you; take time to reflect on it before you respond. Is this person trying to get a reaction out of you? Are the comments true? Are they coming from a good place? When you feel this frustration or stress coming on, it is probably best to put the phone down and go for a run or read a book.

- Pay close attention to your screen time. If it is exceeding an average of one hour per day, reassess what you are doing on your phone and reduce the time you spend on it.

CHECK OUT

Bailey Parnell, 'Is social media hurting your mental health?' (TED Talk)

Schwartz, J. (2016). *Disconnect to connect: Emotional responses to loss of technology during Hurricane Sandy*. In Emotions, Technology, and Behaviors (pp. 107-122). Academic Press.

FOMO and jealousy

Your mates want to check out a new cocktail bar, but you're really not feeling it because you have had a shitty few weeks at work and would rather just spend the day watching a season of *Stranger Things*. You also have a lot of study to get through before your exam next week, but your mates would just tell you to study tomorrow. So, you lie and tell them you cannot make it because you have to pick up your aunty from the airport. You go to scroll through your phone later that night and see all your mates having a blast. Everyone is dancing and having food and drinks which look amazing. You start to feel depressed and sad as you now wish you could turn back the clock and say yes.

All your mates are going to reference the night for a while to come and you are just going to have to laugh it off and pretend it does not bother you.

This is not the first time you have felt this way because you often turn down events like this. Your mental health and busy schedule have taken over your life and forced you to stay at home.

Exams have finished, and you are looking forward to seeing your mates again. However, they organise another event where they do not invite you at all. You start to feel really lonely and wonder if your friends have completely forgotten about you and lost interest in your friendship.

This fear of missing out (FOMO) has a lot to do with the age we live in. Everything is so obtainable and places are a lot easier to get to than ever before. It's also easier than ever to see what everyone else is doing, where they're going and what things they have. This makes us think we can and should have it all in our lives. Seeing these posts can bring on feelings of jealousy. These attractive, smart, adventurous people are living the life that should be yours!

Have you been through that moment when you are on Instagram and came across a post that makes you feel bad about yourself and the life you live? It may be someone travelling the world, buying a house or getting engaged to their high school sweetheart. I'm not saying it's wrong to share your achievements, experiences or shiny new toys on Instagram. It is completely fine and normal to let your friends know about the accomplishments you feel proud of and the things that make you tick. However, we need to realise that people who are posting things, making it look like they are living the dream life, are only showing you their highlight reel. You don't often see someone posting when they are feeling really sad, embarrassed, or when they just want to cry.

It's important to be mindful of identifying when you are feeling down due to FOMO. Anybody posting your ideal life are highly likely to be living a life like most — they catch the train into work, eat their boring packed lunch and make sure they are in bed by ten. Life is supposed to have boring moments; people just don't show you their boring moments in the same way you don't post selfies while you are doing the dishes, or photos of the traffic jams you encounter in your morning commute.

Realise what would actually happen if you went to that party or social event that made you feel FOMO. Would you really enjoy yourself? Would it be any different to previous events? Is this an event that is significant in your life?

Sure, it's good to go to certain events to catch up with mates, meet new people and enjoy yourself — even if it means going to the same dingy bar — but you should not have to push yourself really hard to go somewhere you know will not benefit you.

Put your phone down. Watch a movie with a family member or partner. Read a book. Phone a friend (lock it in Eddie). Play the guitar. Play COD. Just do whatever will help you keep your mind off things.

Finally, appreciate what you have and try to remain present. Be aware of your thoughts, feelings and emotions and look to accept these. Once you have done this, journal three things you are grateful for in that very moment. This process will help you understand your current emotional state. It will help you realise your life is pretty good and you are actually a pretty good person.

Missing out on these events will not define your life. The grass is often greener on your side as you are the one taking care of the garden.

Material things and online shopping

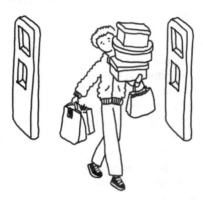

There is always something new that we want to get our hands on. A new phone, dress, shoes, car, cricket bat, tanning product, video game, food or drink. Most companies pump out updated versions of products you probably already own. Why? Companies know the majority of people want to have the most up-to-date product to be perceived as 'trendy'.

We should only be buying things that directly fill a hole in our lives. Yes, there are times when we should treat ourselves or someone we love but this should really only be once in a while.

I have harped on about meditation throughout the book but it is very applicable to this scenario. By taking just 10 minutes of our day to sit with our thoughts and focus on breathing, we are able to bring more rational thinking into our day-to-day lives.

It is wise to take a few days, or even a week, to think about our purchasing decisions. This allows us to assess if we actually need the product. We are then able to assess if the product is going to add more to our current lives and if it will be something we will use regularly over the next few years.

Conduct a stocktake on what you already own. If you have the intention of going to the shops to buy a pair of black jeans, get out all the black jeans you own, if any, and see if the purchase is really necessary. If you can go without a new pair for a few months, it's probably best to keep your money in your pocket.

Are you only buying this thing to impress someone else? For example, do not buy a new car to impress someone from work you fancy; they are not going to think you are a better person just because you spent over $100,000 on a piece of metal.

Shop when you are in a state of calm. When we are stressed, we buy things we do not need as we are more vulnerable to advertising ploys from the large corporations. A young man who is low on confidence due to his struggles dating, might see a deodorant ad and believe this will be the answer to all his problems. It might get rid of his BO but It's unlikely to get rid of his confidence issues.

Declutter your life and throw out things you never wear or have any real use for. Have you taken a look in your room lately and asked, 'Do I actually use or need everything in this room?' This might sound a little crazy but by letting go of things we do not need, we actually gain more. You gain more time by managing less stuff and you gain a sense of freedom by not being controlled by material things.

Nature and the great outdoors

There are definitely benefits to using your mindfulness practice in an outdoor setting.

We know mindfulness puts us in a more positive mood, reduces stress and allows us to be more present.

Being more connected with nature can improve the overall experience of meditation as you are breathing in fresh air, noticing the sounds of nature around you and even catching a bit of sun which is always good for our immune system (if it's a nice day, of course).

You can do meditation in your backyard or at a park where you feel comfortable and will be able to keep your concentration.

The benefits are even there when you are out for a nature walk or stroll. Be aware of the birds, the rustle of the leaves and the cool or hot wind on your body; enjoy all the little things on your walk. It is best to take these walks without any devices; this will keep you focused on the walk and allow you to see how little you actually need technology.

If you have dogs, bring them along for the experience. Notice how much they enjoy being out in nature. Let them off the lead and watch them run around in excitement, showing how happy they are to be out and about. This can lead us to appreciate what we have.

Pets

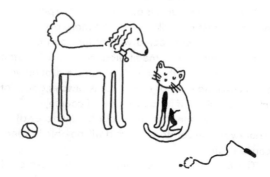

Something that can bring about a more natural and wholesome lift to our mood is loving your pets. You may love your pets so much you want to show pictures of them to everyone you know.

People love their pets for many reasons: their fun and loving nature, the freedom to act as silly as you want around them and, most important of all, pets love their owners unconditionally. Whether you are mean, happy, angry, anxious, depressed or even a little psycho, your pet will never stop loving you.

This is why it is crucial we take time out in our day to be present with them.

If you own a dog, leave your phone at home when you are taking it out for a walk. Be present with your pet and notice how happy it is to be out in nature. Watch your pet run around the park or splash in the water at the beach. You will not be able to stop yourself from smiling.

If you own a cat, sit with them and listen to them purr as you stroke them. Use this as a meditational practice to focus in on your pet's features and emotions — the colour of their eyes, the texture of their fur or coat, whether they are happy or sad. This practice forces you to focus your mind on something you love and can help shift the attention from your own thoughts.

When you are present with your animal companion, notice the happiness you feel thanks to them. It is also important to notice when they are feeling tired or sad. Some dogs will bounce up and down with joy when they sense they are going for a walk, whereas other dogs do not like walks or may simply not be in the mood on a particular day. Whatever the reason, be aware of your pet's emotions and look for other ways to cheer them up if walks aren't their thing.

Owning a pet is a brilliant way of expressing love and affection. It also allows you to become more aware of yourself while also being more aware of the things that are most important in your life. Be grateful for the loving relationship you have with your pet because it is tough to find a human who will love you as much as your animal friend does.

If you don't own a pet, this is fine. You can find love in other ways, including family, a friend, or even someone else's pet!

QUOTES & STORIES

WHAT DO OTHER PEOPLE THINK?

'Look deep, deep into nature, and then you will understand everything better.'

ALBERT EINSTEIN, in a letter to his stepdaughter Margo, 1951

'We are so immersed in an acclimated to the experience of our fast-paced, digital lives that it is challenging to gain a sense of the traumas subtly embedding each day.'

BONNIE BADENOCH, *The Heart of Trauma: Healing the Embodied Brain in the Context of Relationships*

'Exchange your online distractions for real-life devotion.'

WENDY SPEAKE, *The 40-Day Social Media Fast: Exchange Your Online Distractions For Real-Life Devotion*

'Dogs are our link to paradise.'

MILAN KUNDERA, *The Unbearable Lightness of Being*

'The most dangerous distractions are the ones you love, but that don't love you back.'

JAMES CLEAR, jamesclear.com

'An addiction to distraction is the end of your creative production.'

ROBIN SHARMA, *The 5AM Club*

'When I am feeling low all I have to do is watch my cats and my courage returns.'

CHARLES BUKOWSKI, *The Pleasures of the Damned*

'The power and temptations of the outside world are great. Train yourself from the distractions. They are the enemies of your goals. Learn to move past the distractions, and you will succeed.'

JESSE ITZLER, *Living with the Monks: What Turning Off My Phone Taught Me About Happiness, Gratitude, and Focus*

ROBERT DOWNEY JR

Downey was introduced to drugs at the age of six when his dad would allow him to smoke cannabis. Downey and his dad would take drugs together as a way of bonding with one another. He later became addicted to heroin and even spent six months in prison for avoiding a drug test. According to the District Recovery Community: Downey managed to quit drugs in 2001. Downey relied on a number of holistic therapies and filled the void left by his abstinence by taking up yoga and Wing Chun kung fu. He also credits the support he received from his spouse as the source of his success in recovery. Downey is also an advocate of Twelve Step recovery programs.

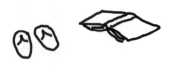

MINDFULNESS
AROUND OTHERS

Listen for once

Daisy and Rose are catching up for their weekly coffee run down at their local. Daisy just recently got sacked from her job, so this meet-up has extra significance. They sit down and Daisy lets everything out — why she got fired, her emotional state and how her world is falling apart around her.

Rose sits there nodding and acknowledging everything Daisy is saying. About halfway through Daisy's spiel, Rose takes a quick glance at her phone and sees a text from her gym friend regarding the time they were planning on doing their boxing class. Rose's attention is now focused on her gym friend. Daisy continues to speak and Rose continues to nod and acknowledge everything Daisy is saying.

What Rose did not realise is she unknowingly said yes to help Daisy with her résumé tomorrow.

The next day, while at her gym class, Rose receives a phone call from Daisy.

'Where are you?'

'At the gym, why?'

Daisy angrily tells Rose they were supposed to meet up today and says she is very disappointed in her. Daisy hangs up. Rose feels terrible. Daisy later starts wondering if Rose was even really listening to her the whole time.

We all zone out of conversations. Especially ones that do not impact us directly. Sure, we love our friends and we would do a lot for them, but some people can find it hard to pay attention for long periods of time.

In this scenario, Daisy had just been sacked. Rose should understand Daisy needs her full attention — she is in a heightened negative emotional state and needs support from her friend. On the other hand, Daisy could have been a little more alert to her friend's cues and seen that Rose's attention was not fully on her.

No blame should be laid on either friend; there was just a lack of awareness and presence from both.

We need to make the conscious effort to listen and make sure we fully understand what others are communicating to us. Not just listening with our ears but seeing the emotions in facial expressions and watching hand movements to capture the true feeling behind what is being said.

We can improve our listening in many ways:

- Empathy — listen from someone else's point of view. If someone is saying something that you do not fully agree with, accept this is their opinion and understand it is not necessarily fact. Do not take it personally. Try to be open-minded to other ways of thinking.

- Practise meditation every day and, if you have to, take a little time to observe your mental state before seeing someone and while you are with them. If you find yourself not listening, calmly bring yourself back to the present moment.

- Do not take any devices with you when you are seeing a friend or, if that's not possible, commit to keeping devices out of reach. 'No phones' should be a rule for your catch-ups with friends.

Some people are just negative

Most of us have encountered at least one negative person in a team or group before—whether through work, school or a sporting team. This person usually managed to bring the mood of everyone else down as they always seemed to be angry or upset over anything and everything. For example, when another team member is getting a lot of recognition, the negative team member may start to gossip about the integrity of the boss or how it should be him getting the praise over the team member getting the recognition.

We need to be mindful of these people. Understand that others may have been brought up differently or have been surrounded by an environment that forces them to think and act in this way. If you feel these negative emotions are being directed at you, try to catch yourself when you feel this way, and know that these unhealthy messages should not be taken personally or as fact.

It may be wise to try to lighten up the situation, perhaps through humour or by changing the discussion topic. By doing this, you are catching the negativity out and will be able to quickly move on from these feelings. You can then focus your energy on something more positive.

If a person is being negative and you can see they are greatly affected by it, check up on them if you feel you are close enough to them to do so. Maybe they are going through some serious issues in their personal life that are taking over their social life outside of home. Checking up on people helps them become aware of their thoughts and emotions and should drive them to reassess themselves and try to find positivity in their life.

It doesn't hurt to keep a smile on your dial. Even if you feel like you are faking it, you may find that by putting on a smile, you are able to work your way through difficult encounters with others in a more positive manner.

You are better than your haters

'What other people think of me is none of my business.'
ELEANOR ROOSEVELT

Not everyone is going to like you. That is just one of the many realities of life.

They may not like you for no good reason. You may be too positive, you may be friends with someone they have bad history with, or it could even be because you did not say 'Hi' to them when you walked past in the staffroom kitchen one time, seven months ago.

This often happens if you are perceived to be a leader in your work life. As a leader, one of your primary focuses is making the right decisions. When these decisions do not go entirely to plan, people may look to ridicule and undermine you. Rumours may start to spread about your ability to fulfil the role. This can lead to more of your team members thinking negatively of you.

People who find themselves to be successful in other ways also face this issue. Haters are often jealous of the way successful people live their lives because everything seems to come easily to them. Or haters may think these successful people do not deserve the accolades and lifestyle they received.

If you find yourself in a situation where other people's perceptions of you are impacting your emotions and overall wellbeing, just remember these perceptions do not define you.

The people who know you on a deep personal level know your values and what you stand for. If you are genuinely someone who wants the best for yourself and everyone around you, those close to you will know you are acting with integrity.

If your job, or any group you are a part of, involves a toxic environment, talk to these people directly or to a leader. If this fails, you always have the option to quit and find somewhere else. You can also block these people on your social media if they are not worth keeping in touch with.

It's important to note that if someone is trying to offer feedback on something you have said or done, you should not consider this a form of hate. Understanding the difference between hate and feedback is vital, especially in this 'cancel culture' society where people are easier to offend than ever before. If it's hate, the tone and the use of words will be more aggressive and unhelpful, compared to a positive, friendlier approach aiming to help. The ability to receive and use constructive criticism to your advantage is crucial for your resilience and growth.

The same can apply to a bit of friendly banter. Jokes and pranks with close friends are often not meant to be hurtful. If you feel personally hurt by something a mate has joked about, write down why you feel this way. You can also write down whether this was a personal attack on you or not. Doing this helps you to better understand and rationalise the kind-heartedness of the joke.

People who are jealous of you only feel this way because they feel miserable about their own life. Haters want to bring you down, as haters love seeing people fail. If you are unable to reason with these people face-to-face, remove them your life. It is important to surround yourself with people who are fully loving and supportive of you.

CHECK OUT

Elizabeth Yuko, 'How to tell the difference between constructive criticism and bullying' in Lifehacker (web article).

Find a mentor

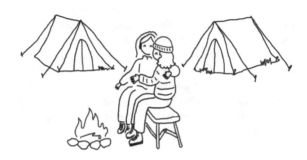

We can often get lost in our adventure through the journey of life. Thankfully, we have wise people, such as our parents, teachers and bosses who are there to guide us and provide us with instructions on how to navigate effectively through our lives.

Mentors can be helpful in our mindfulness practice. When we are in a mental state where we are stuck for answers, we can call on a mentor to provide us with the knowledge and experience to guide us through tough times.

You may have a neighbour, a mate or a family member who has had life experiences that correlate to your current situation. They can help you find the right path without the need to try to seek out a relationship with a totally new person. For some, talking to someone they are fully comfortable with is all they need.

You can even find mentors online – professionals, YouTubers, podcasters and so on. Some of these people are obviously very hard, or impossible, to reach but we do not need to be directly in contact with them to use their knowledge. For example, you may find someone like Russell Brand to be a great mindfulness teacher. He has had his fair share of personal struggles and is now a much more spiritually and mentally aware person.

If you are looking for a more personal relationship with a professional, you can find people online who you can chat to directly. Alternatively, you can go on mindfulness and mental health retreats and share your experiences, fears and aspirations with a group.

A mentor should be available often. Of course, we all have our own schedules we need to live by but if a mentor has agreed to help someone out, they should find time to help when they can. Whether online, by text, a phone call or face-to-face, we are always able to find ways to keep in touch when it's important.

The mentor should be able to see when their mentee is in a heightened emotional state and should adapt their discussion to calmly resolve an issue or provide the mentee with more clarity.

For some, speaking to a certified psychologist can also be very beneficial. Even though this option is usually more expensive, it is often better to speak to a professional to get answers to our questions relating to any mental health or life issues we may be having trouble with.

You can use online sources such as psychology. org.au to find a psychologist who suits your particular needs. In Australia, a certain number of sessions with a mental health professional can sometimes be fully or partially paid for with Medicare. Talk to your GP to see if this, or a similar program, is something you can take advantage of.

Finding someone who you can speak to as openly as possible is crucial to finding clarity and interpreting our thoughts the way they are meant to be treated — as thoughts. The more we talk about our thoughts and difficulties in our life, the less scary they will appear.

You and everyone else are doing their best

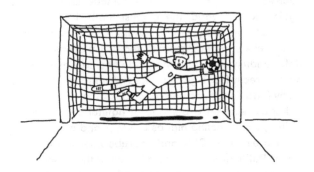

There are certain people who we are naturally intimidated by. Conversations with a boss are usually job-specific, and you may not have spoken to them on a personal level, even after working with them for quite some time. If you were to bump into your boss on the street, would you approach them and say hello or pretend you did not see them and walk in a totally different direction?

You may see a celebrity who has been heavily linked to a scandal in the press. An immediate reaction for some could be to think of this person as one who should be taken down or publicly shamed. Traditional media platforms use someone else's controversy and turmoil to portray a negative narrative in order to get clicks and views for their network. How heartless and messed up is that?

Some people do the same on social media. They give their thoughts on famous and infamous people through platforms, such as Twitter, and hide behind a screen, ripping into someone we have never even had a conversation with.

In 2018, Loris Karius was a young, promising goalkeeper playing for world famous Liverpool FC against Real Madrid, the biggest football club in the world at the time, in the Champions League final. This is every young, aspiring football player's dream. Unfortunately for Karius, he made two crucial mistakes which directly led to goals for Real Madrid. In the eyes of many fans, Karius cost Liverpool the game.

Karius received a barrage of hateful comments on Twitter, disrespecting him as a player and as a person. There are memes, GIFs, and YouTube videos making fun of him. Rational viewers would feel empathy for someone who has to perform at an extraordinarily high standard with the whole world watching them. How would you want people to treat you if you made those mistakes?

Yes, these people get paid the big bucks, but do they really deserve this level of extreme hate when they make mistakes similar to those any of us could make in our own jobs? The difference is — when we make mistakes, not many people know about them.

No matter how mistakes happen, we should be there for people in times where they feel the most shame and embarrassment. It is not as if people deliberately try to do wrong.

For as much hate as Karius copped, he did receive a lot of love from other sportspeople. People came to fight in his corner, including former Real Madrid player, Dani Ceballos who tweeted: 'Lots of encouragement, friend! Football always offers second chances. Let's go!' This just proves that social media can be a platform to provide positive views and support in times of need.

We all do our best to live the life we know we are capable of. We try our best to be kind to others, stay healthy, have a steady income and so on. Everyone is doing the best they can to balance the life they are living and to find their own state of happiness. Next time you have the opportunity to bring someone down, try to lift them up instead.

Don't take everything personally

Most of us have had a disagreement with a friend, a parent or even a teacher at least once in our life. An initial reaction for some may be to verbally attack the other person, often on a deeper, more personal level. Why do we get so defensive over words? Why do we fight back when it's not usually needed?

Try to view these confrontations as chances to improve your mindfulness.

Understand where the other person is coming from. We do not all view the world in the same way. We are all different! Everyone's values and beliefs are different and we usually take different things more or less seriously or personally than others.

If someone is saying something that is hurtful or frustrating, they may have been brought up to act in this way. People who were brought up in negative environments look to bring others down to make themselves feel more superior. They also try to win every confrontation they are part of, even if it means hurting someone they love. It may be the person is trying to have a rational conversation with you, but the way they react to or converse with others is a by-product of how they have been raised or of other circumstances in their life. Try your best to see what is being said from the other person's point of view.

Now you are more aware of the person's background and why they may have attacked you personally, detach yourself from what this person says about you. View these attacks on you as their own unhealthy mindset and upbringing, rather than facts about you. Doing this involves not reacting in a way that indicates you have bitten on their bait — do not yell or get fired up. Try to act as neutral and calm as possible.

It is also important to make sure you understand if the other person is retaliating to something they have perceived to be a personal attack. You can do this by carefully listening to them and thinking back to how the argument started. You can even show compassion for this person. Knowing they are negative can provide you with the chance to check up on them. Maybe they are having a bad week at work. It takes a lot of mental power to remain present in a moment that is so intense, but it can be done.

Catch yourself when you, or someone you are with, is not self-aware. When we are in a heated argument, it is hard to realise we are not acting in a mindful way. Remove or detach yourself from the conversation and ask yourself if the confrontation is really worth it. If you feel the conversation should be revisited because an important issue needs to be resolved, approach this person later in a mindful manner and do your best to calmly resolve the issue.

If someone is consistently behaving in an antagonistic way, consider distancing yourself from the relationship. This person may keep wanting to bait you until you bite. If you find you are involved in relationships similar to this, it may be wise to take a break from them or cut off ties completely, depending on how much you value the relationship.

Friendship and companionship is vital for happiness

Remember how much easier it was making friends when we were young? For some people, making friends at school may have been difficult but for the majority it was easy to just go up to people for the first time, without fear or hesitation, and instantly bond. Imagine trying to do that as an adult.

Adults find it very hard to make friends. We are usually comfortable with the mates we have and are not seeking to make new ones.

Our closest mates are great at picking us up when we feel down, making us laugh until we cry, bouncing ideas around with and sharing life aspirations. We can talk to mates with little to no filter. How great is it to talk crap with someone who really gets you? No need to have that boring old chit-chat about the weather just because it's polite.

Studies show the happiest people are those who are the most social. It is also apparent that friendship reduces stress and lowers our blood pressure, since we feel more relaxed and have less opportunity to overthink. In their work on the relationship between wellbeing and social relationships. Richard Lucas and Portia Dyrenforth state that,

> People who are sociable and extroverted experience more positive affect than those who are not. People who spend more time with others are happier than those who spend a lot of time alone. People who have many friends are happier than those who have only a few. And people who are married are happier than those who are divorced or widowed.

This has a lot to do with not overthinking when interacting with others and being confident in who we are. We can think too much about trying to act cool, making sure we do not offend others or coming across as weird.

In order to stop this overthinking, we need to get out there a lot more. You can build up your confidence by doing the simplest things: ring your local takeaway instead of ordering online, stop and have a conversation with a fellow dog walker or catch up with a mate who you are not super close with.

Once you have built up the self-esteem, you can look to use your experience interacting with others to form new friendships. If your current environment does not allow you to meet new people, consider joining a new social club, gym, art group, or wherever you think you can meet people who share similar interests to you.

By doing this, you will become more confident in yourself which will reflect onto other people and into other areas of your life.

CHECK OUT

Lucas, R. E., & Dyrenforth, P. S. (2006). 'Does the Existence of Social Relationships Matter for Subjective Well-Being?' In Self and relationships: Connecting intrapersonal and interpersonal processes (pp. 254–273). The Guilford Press.

Mayo clinic, 'Friendships: Enrich your life and improve your health' (web article)

Chris Woolston, 'Health benefits of friendship', in HealthDay (web article).

Loneliness

People feel lonelier than they ever have been before. Technology, romantic movies and social expectations have moulded us to not only feel lonelier but to view loneliness as something only a loser goes through.

You may picture a lonely person being someone who cries in their room every night because they have no friends. This may be the case with some but not all.

Loneliness can arise within anyone, including people who are in a committed relationship or have an active social life. These people are often trying to fill the void of loneliness through the love of another person, whether that be a spouse or a friend. You cannot expect someone else to fill the void of loneliness — this needs to be done internally.

It is important to understand why you feel lonely. You may be someone who avoids lonely feelings through trying to stay busy or going on social media. You need to ensure you are giving yourself time to sit with your own thoughts to truly understand why you are feeling lonely. Is it because you want a loving relationship like you see in the movies? Are you jealous of how that guy from work seems to be loved by everyone? Do you just want someone to talk with so you are not left alone with your own thoughts? Whatever the reasons are, you need to make sure you work at this through being present and being more aware of your emotional state. Write down these reasons in your journal. Once you have done this, write down some strategies to tackle these reasons. This may include being more social in your workplace or changing your mindset through meditation and reading. Use mindfulness practices, such as watching your thoughts, without judgement, from an outsider's perspective, or bird's eye view, as they come and go through your mind.

Taking a lone wolf approach to life can also be an effective way of settling these feelings. You may be wondering how being lonely will fix your lonely feelings? Using a lone wolf approach does not mean you can never talk to anyone else ever again, however, taking a risk to be lonely and to learn more about yourself will better equip you to dealing with these emotions. By taking this approach, you will learn more about yourself and understand the things in life that make you feel fulfilled and happy. Try solo travelling, going on walks alone, take up a hobby where you are by yourself, like surfing. The more you immerse yourself in your own thoughts, the more you contextualise these feelings and the better you will be at living with your thoughts day-to-day.

By knowing how to deal with feelings of loneliness and learning more about yourself, you will also allow yourself to feel more love towards you. How can you expect somebody else to love you when you don't love yourself? It is very difficult to connect to another person on a deep and meaningful level if you have doubts about yourself. To connect with someone else, it takes vulnerability. By not being vulnerable, you will tend to be hesitant and hold back on saying things that are truly you. By loving yourself more, you will be able to connect and speak more freely to others as you will become more comfortable with the person you are.

Everyone feels lonely from time to time. Understanding why you feel this way and being able to deal with it and live with your own thoughts is such a powerful way to lessen the impact of these emotions. Keep using mindfulness as a gateway to accept your emotions. Mindfulness has to be used for a long period of time for the habit to well and truly sink in. Set aside time for it! Just remember — at the end of the day, your best friend should always be you.

Make amends with someone you have done wrong by

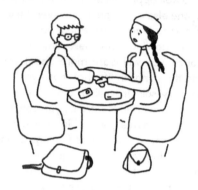

Most close relationships, whether platonic or romantic, will lead to disagreements, betrayal, ridicule, and falling out from time to time. Some relationships are irreparable as one person can go too hard or personal on the other. Disrespecting someone's character, integrity or values can be received very negatively, especially for someone who is vulnerable. When this happens, it is important to know when you have done wrong and apologise.

We are not being mindful when we do wrong by someone. If we knew what we were doing was wrong, we would not do it, right? Well, a lot of us still do wrong by others, even when we are mindful of it; we just choose to go down a road that seems to be either more beneficial or has fewer negative effects on ourselves and those close to us.

There appears to be a stigma around apologising. This is because we are making it known to others that we did something wrong. It is a big hit to our ego. When we are able to separate ourselves from our ego, we are able to accept our wrongs without any negative emotions of shame or guilt attached.

The first thing we should try to do when apologising is to say why we are sorry: 'I'm sorry I couldn't make it to your party.' Even though you may have had a legitimate reason for not making it to the party, you should make it known you are genuinely upset you could not make it and that you ended up hurting someone you care about.

The next thing we should do is to consider the other person's feelings. It is also important to own the mistake and accept responsibility for what we did: 'I know this party meant a lot to you and I should have made more of an effort to make it.'

Finally, we should make amends for what we did: 'Is there anything I can do to make it up to you?' It can be the smallest thing, such as helping with the clean-up the next day. The important thing is showing our mates we value their companionship.

Waiting for an apology, and accepting it, is a skill, too. We don't want to put someone down when they are apologising to us: 'Finally!' or, 'You were such a dickhead for doing that.' The best thing to do is to either accept or decline the apology and move on with the decision you have made in a manner that is respectful to both parties. In saying this, try your best to accept apologies, even if you cannot forget the bad things the person has done to you. Learn to live in the now and see the person for who they are trying to be today.

If you are lucky enough to have the opportunity to make amends with someone you have done wrong by, take the courage to do this. Some relationships can be easily repaired by one person taking the initiative to say they were wrong. Most will accept your apology, especially if it is someone who you have good history with.

Please also refer to the chapter 'Sometimes losing is better than winning' for more on a similar topic.

Compliments and thanks

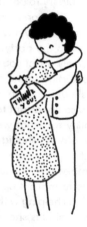

Giving out compliments increases the mood of both the receiver and the giver.

Compliments need to be genuine: only offer them when they are warranted. If you start forcing this and being insincere, the receiver will see right through you.

You can start by complimenting your partner: 'Your hair looks nice today.'

You can give a compliment to someone from work: 'You did a really good job with that customer yesterday.'

If you feel comfortable enough, you can even start complimenting strangers on the street!

Another way of lifting our mood is to thank those who are closest to us.

Write a letter (with a pen) to a mate, a loved one, family member or colleague — anyone who made you feel loved or did something that helped you along your life journey. You may not get the immediate reaction you were looking for but that is not why you are doing this.

This letter will make you feel positive for spreading love and appreciating someone closer to you. This will also strengthen relationships in your life.

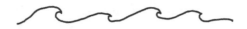

QUOTES & STORIES

WHAT DO OTHER PEOPLE THINK?

'Isn't it kind of silly to think that tearing someone else down builds you up?'

SEAN COVEY, *The 7 Habits of Highly Effective Teens*

'The strong-minded rise to the challenge of their goals and dreams. The weak-minded become haters.'

STEVE MARABOLI, *Unapologetically You: Reflections On Life and The Human Experience*

'It's not a person's mistakes which define them – it's the way they make amends."

FREYA NORTH, *Chances*

THE BEATLES

In the 1960s, The Beatles got rejected by Decca Records. Their reason for rejecting the band was supposedly that 'guitar groups are on the way out'.

MANAGING
DIFFICULT
EMOTIONS AND
SITUATIONS

Media

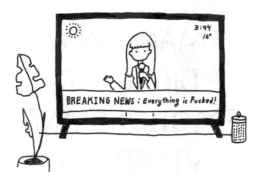

News sources love to flood us with information. Yes, it is important to stay informed about what is going on in the world, but when we consume too much information, we can begin to feel overwhelmed.

We start to believe anything we hear – the world is going to end due to low water supply, global hunger, corruption or even a pandemic.

News media companies use their platforms to persuade the audience. We become stressed and anxious because we are fearful about what is going to happen in the future or what is currently going on in the world.

They often use clickbait titles and pictures in a bid to persuade us to click to their website.

We also become a lot more judgemental about things we do not fully understand. We can become biased toward certain media outlets or to the most recent piece of news we hear. Certain media platforms look to provide us with filtered information in order for them to satisfy the network or an external party that might exert influence on them.

It is important to take everything you hear and read with a grain of salt. Don't take every piece of news as fact. Use news platforms you trust, and that you know are reputable. Make sure you read multiple reliable sources and develop your own opinion. A good source to use is Gapminder. They are a foundation whose aim it is to provide reliable and easy to interpret data for people who want to know more about global and economic trends. Check out their website or the TED Talk by founder Hans Rosling.

Try not force your opinion down other people's throats. If you are discussing a news topic with a mate and you believe they are wrong or hold an opinion that is based on clickbait 'fake news' articles, calmly ask why they think this about the topic, and provide your opinion. If they disregard it or talk you down, try not to fight back. This person will most likely not change their mind.

CHECK OUT

Hans Rosling, 'The best stats you've ever seen' (TED Talk).

Gapminder, https://www.gapminder.org/

Find your happy place in dark times

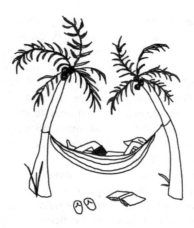

The world is a mad place. There is so much going on around us and we are trying our hardest to keep up. We can often get stuck in a slump where we constantly feel down or let things overwhelm us.

We face daily challenges that can result in increased levels of stress and anxiety, including being stuck in traffic, trying to meet deadlines at work or dealing with difficult family members.

At times like these, we need to realise why we are getting caught up in these emotions. Do we feel how we feel because we will be late to work? Will we rush the work project, and mess it up? Or will we upset family members?

When we begin to feel overwhelmed by life, we need to find our happy place.

You may have heard people on TV or in movies say, 'Go to your happy place' or 'Just think happy thoughts.'

This is often hard to do when we are not in the right frame of mind.

Before you get to your happy place, you will need to practise basic mindfulness techniques.

You can start by changing your lifestyle habits. Leave for work earlier if you are worried about being late. Talk to your boss about needing more assistance for the project or task. Stop holding grudges or stretching out fights with family members. These sound like obvious things to do but it is hard to remind ourselves to do them when we are constantly caught up in our own thoughts. This is where a tool such as diary writing can be of great use. You can note down your problems and work out solutions. Doing this will help calm your mind and reduce any negative emotions you may be holding.

Once you have calmed your mind and changed your lifestyle habits, look to find time in your day to enter your happy place. This practice will take place in the mind, obviously. Close your eyes, count ten breaths, in and out. Then, focus your attention on entering a place that makes you happy. This place can be a nature walk, grabbing a coffee with a mate, going for a run, pursuing a hobby, sailing, a family memory — anything that makes you happy. Once your mind is in this place, try to live it as much as you can and spend as much time there as you need. Feel the sunshine on your face and listen to birds chirping or the waves crashing.

This practice is a form of visualisation and is used by a lot of athletes before they go into a game or event. They picture moments that are likely to happen in a game — often moments of difficulty. By visualising these moments before they happen, they can prepare their mind and body for what is to come and be ready for it. We can also do this in our happy place or during meditation time. Think of a moment you expect to happen with a boss or family member and try to visualise yourself communicating and reacting to this person in a calm and calculated manner.

Do what works for you. You can do this anywhere you feel safe and have privacy. If your workspace is too busy or chaotic, consider taking a quick bathroom break to get away for a few moments.

If you start to do this every day, or even just on days you know you will feel stressed, you will be amazed at how much your mindset changes when it faces everyday difficulties.

Being uncomfortable more often

A lot of people like to go through life playing it safe. We may avoid confrontation, things that are challenging and potentially embarrassing situations. We may think we are safe when we live life in this way, but we're more mentally unsafe than we realise.

Uncomfortable experiences are what define the human experience. If you breeze through every challenge or test that comes your way in life, are you really living life the way it is meant to be lived?

Think of something we talked about in a previous chapter — your favourite TV character, for example. Are you watching the show because you are interested in how super easy the characters' lives are? Or are you watching because you find their lives relatable and are intrigued to see how they deal with life's ups and downs?

A lot of uncomfortable moments would have occurred during your school years, such as giving a speech in front of the class, talking to someone who you liked or going on a school camp. You may look back at some of these moments with guilt or embarrassment because you ran away from the moment or did something silly.

Learn how to be comfortable with your uncomfortable thoughts and emotions.

Whatever it was that you did, consider how it has shaped you today. When you encounter uncomfortable situations in the future, you will be much better equipped. You will be prepared to deal with that sick feeling in your stomach, shortness of breath or your heart pounding in your chest. The more uncomfortable experiences you confront, the more you begin to understand your world is not going to end because of these challenging moments.

You may become uncomfortable through over-thinking. You may have a big event coming up or feel ashamed of something you have done in your past. To keep your mind occupied and avoid these thoughts, you may try to be as busy as you can by over-exercising or doing housework all day. It is important to take time out of your day to sit with your thoughts, whether it is through your meditational practice or, when you have time in your day, just sitting in silence.

We do not need to be happy with these thoughts, just accepting of them. We are not attacking these thoughts or strangling them until we feel no pain from them at all. We want to let them in, offer them a drink and see what they have to say. You will most likely feel uneasy during this practice. Dark thoughts may come and go, but you will learn how to deal with them rather than running away.

Another practice you can take up is immersing yourself in your discomfort. Prioritise maybe two or three things that make you feel sick to your stomach and look to jump into these moments. For example, if you feel nervous about talking to a colleague from work, start by asking them a simple question: 'Where is the boss?' or 'Hey, do you know what time the meeting is today?' Accept this will feel uncomfortable and mistakes are likely to happen. Learn from your mistakes and catch yourself out if you are avoiding situations you know you can handle. Once you start doing this, you will begin to throw yourself into uncomfortable situations without even thinking of them.

Learn to let life unfold the way it was meant to. If we avoid difficult times, this can lead to a numb life. Get out of your comfort zone and watch yourself grow into who you know you can be.

Family

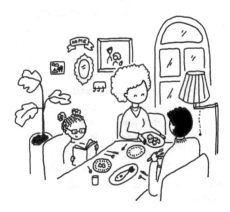

Family always comes first. If this is true, why do we argue with our siblings and disregard lessons our parents teach us?

You may have a brother or sister who annoys you from time to time — or all of the time. They push your buttons for their own entertainment. You get mad and retaliate in a way that ends up getting you both in trouble. Mum and Dad may find it best to discipline both of you in an aggressive manner so you both learn your lesson. You go to your room in a sulk.

These days we look back on those times as character-building experiences. It does not mean these experiences need to happen for us to grow. In order to reduce conflict in the average home, we need to change the environment we all live in. We are not saying go with a laissez-faire or 'hippy' approach, just minor alterations.

Living under the same roof with the same people often leads to others getting on your nerves. It is important to give each other space and privacy. Give everyone their own room where they can escape to — this also applies to Mum and Dad. It does not mean sleeping in different beds but to have a space in the house where you can pursue a passion or relax without being disturbed.

Listen to your family members' concerns with intent. You are not truly taking in what someone is saying when you are flicking through Facebook and Instagram. Put the phone and any other distractions down and focus on who is in front of you and what they have to say. When listening, be present. A good way to do this is to ask questions: 'Why did they do that?', 'What happened next?' and 'How does that make you feel?'. This will ensure you stay engaged in the conversation and your family members will feel like you value what they are saying. This is vital in helping our family through difficult times.

Never be afraid to ask if someone is okay. It may be scary to ask this, especially when you think they will react negatively.

Spend valuable time together. Allocate time in the week to have some fun with your loved ones. Adding family rituals can be really beneficial, for example, going to the footy with your sister/brother every week. Rituals like these create memories that will last a lifetime and allow our bonds with family members to grow stronger.

It is important to have fun together. Have a movie night, a games night, go bowling — whatever gets your family laughing and joking around with each other.

Surprise your mum or dad with a gift once in a while. Your parents do so much for you and have made you the person you are today. Buy them something that could bring them to tears of joy. You will make yourself a lot happier too.

Don't hold grudges. If you have been coming to blows with a brother or sister, apologise — even if you weren't wrong. Life is too short for enemies, especially ones who live under the same roof as you.

You can't choose your family, however you should still try to be thankful for the one you have got as some people don't have a family at all. Even if you do not have the best relationship with your family, try to tell them you love them and you are grateful for how they have shaped you today.

Positivity and gratitude

*'When you are grateful, fear disappears and
abundance appears.'*
TONY ROBBINS

Saying things like 'everything is fine' is not a sustainable
approach to maintaining positivity in your life. Everything
in life is not fine; we all go through our ups and downs.
That said, a positive mindset can help us get out of
any slump.

Pay attention to what is good in your life and be
mindful of those things. Don't focus on what is wrong.
There is too little time to dwell on mistakes and bad
things that have happened in the past.

Being positive isn't just a trick of the mind that makes
you think things are better. Studies show positive
thoughts actually decrease the chances of poor health
outcomes, such as cardiovascular disease and cancer.
You'll find others respond more positively to you if you
have an optimistic outlook, too, which will make social
situations genuinely less stressful and more enjoyable.

A lot of us would be familiar with the 'golden rule'
from childhood: If you don't have something nice to
say, don't say anything at all. Try to use more positive
language in everyday life. This sounds easy but it is not.
It requires us to be more aware of our language and, like
everything else, it takes practice. You can start building
your awareness muscle by noticing when you are about
to say something negative, or a negative thought comes
to your mind.

Avoid using phrases such as 'I can't' and 'I shouldn't'.
Change your wording with people and yourself. You
will then see how your mindset becomes more positive
over time.

Examples of this include: 'Once I make changes to
my schedule, I will be able to spend more time with my

family', 'I will discuss with my boss what things I need to improve on to get that promotion', 'I am going to start going for a morning run to kickstart my day' or 'Zach got a new haircut, I am going to tell him it suits him'.

A common example is when someone in a work meeting comes up with an idea that, in your opinion, could have a potentially negative outcome for the company. In this scenario, you need to process how this person's idea makes you feel — Mad? Annoyed? Confused?

Acknowledge your instant negative reaction and try to offer some positive feedback and constructive criticism in a way where you are not undermining the other person but still being fair and constructive: 'Yes, I can definitely see where you are coming from here. This idea has positives that could benefit the company. However, it is important we think about the outcome if Scenario A and Scenario B happened. We just need to make sure the company is considering every possible scenario. We can discuss this after the meeting at a more convenient time.'

Take some time to smile

Take a moment to pause your life and other obligations to focus on the good that is happening right in front of you. An example could be when you're out and about with your mates and having a great time. Pause and try your best to live in the moment as much as you can.

When you take the time out to meditate, include a smile in your practice. You will find you will begin to smile more in your regular life. Through taking part in this practice, you will find yourself smiling in your social life and at work, leading people to being more attracted to you. This effect is backed up by a 2017 study conducted by Wang et al, who found that 'positive affective displays, such as smiles, lead to positive interpersonal judgements'.

Gratitude journals and affirmations are great tools to use when we are trying to remind ourselves to be positive. Set aside some time every day to write down things you are grateful for and some affirmations that can remind you of good things you have done and are doing with your life.

Read a positive book or watch a positive TV show to help you to feel good. You will discover new ways of finding positivity in your life through other people's successes and stories. I would recommend staying clear of horror movies for this particular practice.

Keep positive people around you. Most of us have a mate who can bring us down when we see them. Hang out with people who look to grow themselves, whether through love, positivity, work, health or other ways. Find people you can share ideas with and help one another out with your growth journeys.

As mentioned earlier by taking on a more positive mindset, you end up attracting more people towards you. You will be more likely to make friends, get the job you are after and inspire other people because your energy will resonate with other people, making them feel good too.

We don't have to be the bubbliest person in the room and jump around like everything in the world is great. We just need to try to twist negative thoughts into positive reinforcements to make ourselves, and others around us, feel better.

CHECK OUT

Kim, E. S., Hagan, K. A., Grodstein, F., DeMeo, D. L., De Vivo, I., & Kubzansky, L. D. (2017). *Optimism and Cause-Specific Mortality: A Prospective Cohort Study.* American Journal of Epidemiology, 185(1), 21–29. https://doi.org/10.1093/aje/kww182

Wang, Z., Mao, H., Li, Y. J., & Liu, F. (2017). *Smile Big or Not? Effects of Smile Intensity on Perceptions of Warmth and Competence.* Journal of Consumer Research, 43(5), 787–805. https://doi.org/10.1093/jcr/ucw062

Panic attacks and being overwhelmed

Count your breaths. Take one big breath in (count 1) and hold for 3 seconds. Let it out until you cannot breathe out anymore (count 2). Breathe in again (count 3). Do this until you reach ten. Repeat the process until you start feeling calm and in the present moment.

Panic attacks are a physical manifestation of severe anxiety in which your body's fight-or-flight mechanisms are triggered, even though there may not be any external threat present. You may experience pain in certain areas of your body, shortness of breath or tightness in your chest. You might feel light-headed or dizzy and start shaking and sweating. This intense feeling makes you think you are helpless and there is no way of controlling it.

You are not going to die!

It may seem like you are experiencing a never-ending struggle, but panic attacks do not last very long. They usually take no more than half an hour, with the worst of the symptoms all happening within the first ten minutes.

With the right approach, you will have the tools ready to help calm down any attack you feel arising.

Do little things to move yourself back into the present moment. Examples include taking a mindful shower and feeling the warm water flow on each part of your body; going for a nature walk and counting every tree or bird you see; using your index finger to stroke each finger of your other hand; or going to your happy place. Experiment and find what works best for you.

Find a close friend to help you through the panic attack. Catch up with this person and find a place to chat. Let them know you experience panic attacks and ask if they can help you when needed. Explain to them what happens when an attack arises, including pains and tightness, and the types of reassuring comments they can say, such as 'You are safe', 'Come back to the present', 'I am here to help'. This will give you give you much needed support and will help you to feel you are not alone.

Let go and forgive yourself. Do not fight against it. The more you try to fight off the attack, the stronger it will become. It is okay to go through difficult moments, no one is perfect. Accept the experience and learn from it. Seeing it as a growth experience will allow you to see anxiety in a less intimidating way.

If this is something that seems to keep happening, it would be a good idea to see a therapist or other mental health specialist. Having an experienced outsider's perspective can be extremely beneficial in finding new ways to approach oncoming attacks. If you are concerned about seeing someone due to the stigma or you think it will not work for you, rest assured it is a normal and healthy thing to do. Although they may not talk openly about it, you probably know several people who are attending regular therapy appointments. Think of it in the same way as an athlete going to get treatment for a hamstring injury or you going to the GP for a sore throat. There's really nothing to lose, so go to your GP, get a referral and try it out. It may change your life.

CHECK OUT

Better Health Channel, 'Panic Attack' (web article).

Beyond Blue, 'Panic Disorder' (web article).

Health Direct, 'Mental health treatment plan' (web article).

Mental Health Foundation Australia (website).

Trauma, shame and embarrassment

Trauma is a very sensitive subject. Trying to understand and feel for someone going through trauma is impossible — everyone's experiences and their reactions to these experiences are different.

Trauma usually consists of feeling overwhelmed by experiences from our past where we feel ashamed or afraid, or ones we simply do not want to revisit. People who deal with trauma experience a crisis-like emotional state where they feel a high level of tension and stress. Sufferers can feel in a vulnerable state and often be in a constant fight-or-flight mode.

Our lives can be greatly shaped from trauma, particularly when we experience something at a younger age. We are vulnerable and unable to process how or why this event happened.

Some traumas can even be as a result of seemingly smaller moments or disappointments in your life, such as failing an exam or being cheated on. These can have a much bigger impact on us than we think.

Some people do not even realise they are suffering from trauma. You may be having moments when you are angry, sad or nervous and not realise these emotions may be triggered from an experience in your past that is not clearly aligned with your current emotions.

What we need to try to understand is that the emotional wounds we carry from our past do not need to cause us pain for the rest of our lives.

Mindfulness can be a close ally in fighting the effects of trauma. It makes sense because a lot of trauma is the result of being stuck in your hurtful past. However, there are occasions where people who use mindfulness meditation encounter trauma that was not previously brought to the surface. These people can also feel humiliated and distressed because they feel worse than before they took up mindfulness practices.

We need to learn to stay and accept our experiences. The practice should have a focus on staying with these moments when we feel comfortable but also trying to bring our attention back to the present moment. By doing so you will also start to build more self-compassion and be kinder to yourself for your past experiences.

Of course, if you feel overwhelmed when staying with a particular memory or moment, try to take a step back from this by going for a walk or hanging out with a mate. Your overall wellbeing is always the most important priority.

It also helps to view these experiences from a 'bird's eye' view. Learn to dissociate yourself from these memories. By doing so, you can look back on these experiences and see them as something not caused by yourself but by someone else entirely. We can find embarrassing things funnier or not as serious when they happen to someone else.

A lot of our shame and trauma is brought about from memories — ones that may not even be factual. A lot of our memories are experiences we thought happened. You may have performed a speech in front of the class and felt super embarrassed due to a mistake you made. You may have thought everyone saw this mistake and now thinks lesser of you. In reality, it's likely no one noticed and, if they did, no one would think twice about it.

We can even edit these memories — put a different voice on, add different characters, change the mood. Train your mind to view these memories in a way that makes it more comfortable for you.

Basic mindfulness does not work for everyone but it can work for most people when modifications are made to ensure people who suffer with trauma can approach the practice in a safe way. It will take time but keep learning, keep experimenting and keep asking questions until you find what is right for you.

If you need help learning how to use your meditation in a trauma-sensitive manner, look to a professional for advice. Preferably someone who specialises in trauma.

Please refer to the chapter 'Shame and guilt from your past' for more on a similar topic.

Our triggers are all different

The way someone speaks, a certain street or shop we drive past, a story from the past that someone is retelling—a comment can be completely random and mean no harm but something about it can stir us up.

It can instantly turn a fairly normal day into a terrible one.

We react differently to these triggers as each of them brings back a different personal issue. Trauma is usually a major fuel source for a trigger when we see something that reminds us of a terrible experience that happened in our past.

Triggers are very personal and can cut us deeply, making us feel great shame, guilt, fear, embarrassment, anger or a host of other emotions.

It is important to identify our triggers and understand why they set us off. We have the ability to control these emotions and how we react.

Make a list of all your triggers in a journal. Note down what your emotions are, what you see, what you hear, what scenarios come up and anything else that springs to mind when you experience any of your triggers.

Use daily meditation and visualisation to help calm your mind and put yourself into situations where you may become triggered. This may require you to take your mind to scenarios of discomfort as you should try to feel the same emotions you experience when you're in these difficult situations.

If someone is saying something in a tone or manner that triggers you, try to understand their situation before reacting. You may be out to lunch with someone from work. You are not best mates with this person but close enough with them to go for lunch. You are both sitting down at the table and you notice your colleague has a scar on the side of his head. Thinking a cool story may come out of this, you ask, 'How did you get that scar?'

Your workmate says, in an embarrassed tone, 'Just fell off my bike as a kid.' He tries his best to cover up the scar and jumps to his feet. 'Oh shit, I've got a meeting in five minutes. See you back at the office.'

You sense this is unusual behaviour, as he would have told you if he had a meeting during lunch. Asking about the scar may have been a trigger for your workmate. This could have forced him to think of a traumatic childhood experience.

The best thing to do in such a situation is ask if your workmate is okay, apologise and say you are there for them if they need somebody to talk to.

These mindfulness tools will help provide some clarity for our triggers. We begin to understand these triggers, make any necessary changes and discover how to best prepare ourselves for triggers we may face in the future. As we grow our awareness, we grow our ability to respond to these triggers in a positive way.

Check in on yourself

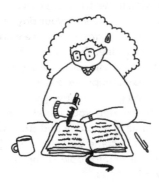

Do you ever wonder how or why you reach a state of heightened anxiety or depression? We spend so much of our energy trying to maintain our own life, we often forget to take the time to check up on how we are feeling. With a lot of us, these questions are asked a little later than we'd like.

This is why it is important to hit pause on your life as often as you can.

This means stepping back from your life and asking yourself questions to better understand your own emotional state.

'Am I okay?'

'Is there anything getting me down, angry or upset?'

'Is there anything making me happy?'

'Am I excited for anything?'

'Is there something in my life that needs changing?'

'What thoughts come into my mind?'

'Am I seeing any visions or bad memories?'

In that moment, when we check in, our attention steers away from the constant commentary in our mind, allowing us to take a look at our emotions through a different lens. Asking these questions can be a great way of assessing where you are with your day or where you want to be long term. We are able to see what is making us happy and sad in life. By noticing and identifying what is affecting us emotionally, we are able to make necessary changes to improve our wellbeing and be grateful for anything good we have going on.

You can do this during your meditation or through journalling. Find time in your day and start by doing this once a day. As you become accustomed to journalling, you might be more comfortable doing it only once a week. Make it work for you.

You can do it on the drive to work or during a boring meeting. Just make sure that when you have thoughts distracting you from your 'check in' work, gently come back to the present and back to the practice.

Being accepting of life

It is impossible to avoid the ups and downs of life. If we were happy all the time, things would start becoming dull. Moments of happiness are all the more valuable for the contrast they offer from more difficult times.

When you feel discomfort, whether through tension, pain in your body or negative feelings, learn to pay attention to these sensations. Put a name to the feelings to bring them to the surface. For example, tightness in the chest can be 'anxiety' or 'stress'. By labelling these emotions, we shine a light to them, which allows us to look into these feelings with kindness and understanding.

Notice happy moments — catch-ups with mates or pursuing a hobby you are passionate about. In the same way as when we notice bad experiences, shining a light on our positive life moments can enhance our wellbeing while giving us something to look back on when we find ourselves in a negative emotional state.

When we are accepting of our experiences, we are not fighting against them; we are allowing ourselves to view these moments with a kind and open mind. The more we try to fight against negative emotions, the stronger they will manifest.

By acknowledging thoughts and feelings as being temporary, we are able to avoid these hurtful emotions from prolonging and taking over our lives.

Not everyone has a map that clearly outlines where their life is taking them. If you feel you are lost and not sure how to deal with your emotional state, just focus on taking small steps forward. There will definitely be times where you face adversity and it is often impossible to prepare for these moments. Accepting life for what it is provides us with some effective tools to battle life's big challenges. By implementing this habit into your day-to-day life, you will soon start seeing yourself going along the path to a mindful existence.

You are braver than you think

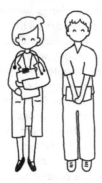

'Bravery is being the only one who knows you're afraid.'
FRANKLIN P JONES

Most likely, not being scared was a big deal when you were a kid. Some of us may have gone to extreme lengths to show how fearless we were. Similar aspects of this can apply to adulthood. You want to give off the vibe to everyone else that you are not terrified of going to that work meeting, or you are as cool as a cucumber working on the 50th storey of a building for a construction company.

You do not need to skydive or go swimming with sharks to think of yourself as brave. Everyone's fears are different, so attack life in a way that suits your means.

Joining a club where you have to fit in among a crowd that has established friendship groups can be an incredibly brave thing to do. Making new friends is hard but if you are just yourself, people will be attracted to you as you will be perceived as authentic.

Leaving your cosy job to start your own business can be a gigantic leap of faith — especially if you are responsible for supporting your family. If you are truly passionate about the idea of working your own hours or starting a job that will satisfy you mentally, take that leap if your research and life situation allow you to.

Sticking to a routine is an example of bravery. If you plan to go for a run every morning, actually doing it not only takes discipline but also a lot of courage.

You may have a medical condition or other issue that prevents you from living a 'normal' life. For example, as a person who has a stutter, I found speaking to strangers incredibly challenging as I felt embarrassed and judged for doing something as simple as ordering a coffee from a cafe. I now understand that my stutter is just a part of my personality and something that should be embraced. These days, I try to live in a way where I never avoid interactions with others to prove to myself that I can overcome my fears.

If you have friends or family who are displaying bravery in their day-to-day lives, look to provide them with words of encouragement and congratulate them for overcoming the challenges they regularly have to encounter, whether they're showing bravery in their work or trying something new, like joining a sporting team. Look to do the same for occasional acts of bravery as well, such as a speech in front of the class.

There are few better feelings in the world than being recognised for your courageous act. Knowing that what you are trying to overcome is something to be congratulated for makes trying to conquer your fears a little easier to bear.

It is also important to know you may never be appreciated for the bravery you display. A lot of doctors never get the recognition they deserve. They have to work in a field that arguably carries the highest stakes. Some doctors can work up to eighty hours a week. When a doctor has done their job by successfully treating someone and, as a result, saved their life, the doctor may be thanked only by the patient and their close family. Why is it rare to hear about these heroic feats on the news? You are more likely to hear about a new bar opening in the city. It was great to see doctors, nurses and other medical staff being appreciated during the COVID-19 pandemic but this gratitude should be shown every day, no matter what is going on in the world.

Getting back on topic, in situations where you feel your bravery is not being recognised by others, learn to congratulate yourself for your heroic feats. Give a little fist pump if you smashed your weight loss goal for the week, treat yourself to a wine or beer if you faced your fear of flying, or play some celebratory music if you went for that job interview. You cannot always rely on others to give you a pat on the back. You should be focusing on feeling good about who you are and what you have achieved.

It is important to be mindful of when you are showing courage in your life. At the end of your week, make notes of all the times you faced your fears. They could be small or large, but you will be surprised how many you will think of. The more things you can get down, the more confidence you will gain as your list can be used as proof that you can face any fear you set your mind to.

Love and heartbreak

If you are on a quest for true love, it is almost certain you have fallen in love or had your heart broken at least once in your life.

Some of us gain the perspective of love through movies and literature, like The Notebook and Romeo and Juliet. These stories can encourage us to perceive love in a way that does not usually correlate to real life.

A lot of people don't end up with the fairy-tale love story; this is just something we need to accept.

Most of us will go through the stages of seeing someone for a long time, to seeing multiple people, then seeing no one for a while.

When we fall in love, we get this feeling of great excitement. You cannot wait to see them and you want to learn more about them. Love is so powerful and is one of the best feelings you can experience. This is why heartbreak can be so devastating when it occurs.

A breakup can mean that you go from hanging out with and talking to this person all the time, to having zero interaction with each other.

We take this heartbreak so personally – often seeing it as a defeat: 'What did I do wrong?', 'Why does this person not want to be with me?', 'Was it something I said?', 'Was I too keen?' or 'Should I have been more open?'.

These questions can lead us to insult ourselves: 'I am ugly', 'I am fat', 'I am not smart enough' or 'I am such a fuck-up'.

We sit with this pain, often for months or sometimes years, replaying moments in our heads and feeling intense emotions, including sadness and anger. This often results in loss of sleep and falling into unhealthy habits. Sometimes we hear a song that reminds us of that person, instantly making us sad again.

This vicious cycle we put ourselves through can be a dangerous place for us to stay in.

The big question we should be asking is: Why do we think our heartbreak is our fault? A lot of accusations and hurtful words can be thrown around in a breakup, and we may end up taking them personally, feeling self-pity as well as increased anger towards the other person. Don't allow yourself to play the victim. It is helpful to realise the breakup that was initiated by the other person is not your fault. You may have thoughts, such as 'Was it something I said or did?' or 'I am not good enough'. A breakup should never be taken as a personal attack on you. Yes, things will be hard at first as you start to remember what it is like to be single and without your best friend. This is when you need to keep taking positive steps forward with your life and recognising you are more than the sum of your relationships.

In saying this, we should allow ourselves to feel these emotions rather than running away from them. Allow yourself to cry or scream into a pillow – there's no point trying to fool yourself that everything is okay when it obviously isn't.

Grab your journal again. Every day, write down the emotions you feel and the thoughts that are racing in your mind. This practice will allow you to process the triggers of your emotional pain and can provide some much-needed perspective for your thoughts.

Over time, as you come to accept your feelings, you can try writing a letter to yourself or the person who broke your heart. Try not to use a template or copy an example from the internet; it is important to write in a way that is authentically you. The letter does not need to be sent, it can be kept with you or thrown in the bin (like this book if you still feel it might not be for you... the option is always open...), the important thing is that you write down what you really want to say on paper. This process should help you let go of any baggage and provide some closure on your unsuccessful relationship.

Try your best to move on, even if this means downloading Tinder again. Get back on the horse, because the worst thing we can do is expect our ex to be waiting for us.

Remind yourself you are good enough. When we are in such a dark emotional place, we often forget the areas of our lives that we are proud of. Make a list of these things or learn how to best revisit these moments. It could be as simple as playing your favourite instrument or spending time in your garden. We can also apply this to our mindfulness meditation through using words of wisdom to help us realise our worth: 'I am good enough' or 'I am worthy'.

Podcasts and YouTube videos based on love and heartbreak allow you to listen to the views of another person and help us find new tactics to deal with our heartbreak.

It is important to note that romantic love, or lack of it, is not necessarily something that will define your life. If you are single and thinking that perhaps you are not sure you want to find love, this can be great for you. As long as you plan out what you wish to get out of your life, then love is something that does not need to be prioritised.

If you do find love, learn from your past mistakes and try your best to be present in the good times. We want our relationships to be remembered for the good times, so by staying present we will not only remember these times with fondness, but we will be a lot happier in the moment.

Crying

We all cry, for many reasons — perhaps we feel stressed and overwhelmed from work or school, grief over death, failed love, or relief and pride for achieving something incredible we have worked so hard for.

A lot of people try to hold back their tears, especially in public, as it may be seen as a sign of weakness. It is important to listen to your body during stressful times. If we allow ourselves to cry, we will learn more about ourselves and become a lot more resilient.

Crying allows us to let go and release all the pent-up stress we are holding onto. If we refuse to let ourselves cry, we will only become increasingly stressed over time.

It is weird that we can cry for both happy and sad moments. According to neuroscientist Jordan Gaines Lewis, our brains cannot always differentiate negative and positive emotions. This can lead to our brain telling us to cry as a way of soothing us when we are overwhelmed with any type of emotion. This is why we can sometimes get teary over seeing a really cute baby or dog.

You may not want to get into a relationship or take on a life journey that you feel will in some way hurt you. Do not let the fear of tears stop you from living life!

Don't fear the tear!

Next time you have a moment when you need to cry, try your best to be in that moment. Think about what has triggered you and why these emotions have come about. You can then write these down in a journal as a reminder of your triggers and how to be more accepting of them.

CHECK OUT

Jordan Gaines Lewis, 'Why do we cry when we're happy?' in *Psychology Today* (web article).

Music

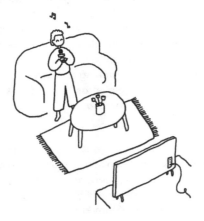

Music is such a powerful tool when it comes to evoking certain emotions. People often listen to love songs after heartbreak, pump-up songs before going to the gym or chilled-out songs when chatting away with mates at a barbecue.

Music can be a great alternative to bring mindfulness into our day-to-day lives.

The ways you can do this include:

Learning an instrument

No matter which musical instrument you are interested in, playing an instrument allows you to be aware of multiple areas of your body. Your eyes, ears and hands are often intertwined to create a particular sound. When you are playing, try to focus on the sounds you are producing. Are the sounds loud? Low or high in pitch? Aggressive? This process will keep your mind focused on something meaningful while growing your awareness muscle.

Using mindfulness music within our practice

When we meditate, we can use a guided meditation to help us through the practice. Try using mindfulness music every so often to spice up your daily meditation. This music involves calming sounds, including waves, nature and chilled techno. You can easily find mindfulness music on Spotify or YouTube. Listening to music is a great way of finding your happy place, as music and sound can take us back to good times in our lives.

Sing

Go into your room, the longue room, the shower, wherever it is and belt out a few of your favourite tunes. If you decide to share the experience with family or mates, it is a great way of getting everyone out of their shell. If you wish to do some private karaoke or sing into your hairbrush when no one is home, this is still a great way to vent out any frustration and get you back in a good mood. It is especially encouraged if you are a rubbish singer!

Music is great for keeping your mindfulness practice fresh. You will have days when sitting in a quiet room is not going to inspire you to use mindfulness or to meditate. Music or sounds may help you find presence and calm through a completely different, and often enjoyable, platform

Believe, love and be kinder to yourself — Billy's story

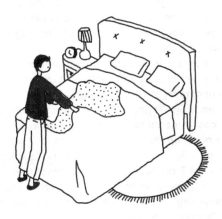

Billy, 23, has recently finished his degree and has picked up a part-time job as journalist for a local newspaper.

It's Sunday night and Billy is lucky enough to be doing a podcast the next day with some reputable journos in the industry. This could be a big step up for Billy and a great way to launch his career.

After doing all his prep for the podcast, Billy receives a message from his mates asking him to come out for a few 'Sunday sippas'. Billy tells them he has a big day tomorrow, so he has to turn it down.

About an hour later, Billy receives another message from one of his mates: 'Sophie just rocked up! Are you sure you still don't wanna come?'

Sophie is a girl Billy has been keen on for a while now. The two have been talking a little but Billy has always been too nervous to ask her out on a date.

Billy negotiates with himself and decides to go for just one drink. He arrives to a big cheer from his mates and sees Sophie at the bar with a few of her friends. Tonight is the night he is going to ask her out on that date.

He approaches and nervously starts talking. Billy can barely get a word out. When he finally manages to drop the question – she turns him down.

Billy returns to his mates in a shattered state. He feels incredibly embarrassed. He goes on a rampage of drugs and alcohol to try to numb the pain.

Billy ends up staying out until 6 am, keeping in mind his podcast is meant to start in three hours.

With no sleep, Billy gets home and instantly crashes on his bed with the intention of having a 'quick nap'. He wakes up at 2 pm to a flood of text messages from the podcasters: 'Ready to go for today?', 'Let us know if you need anything', 'Two minutes to go, are you ready?', 'Billy?', 'Is everything ok?'.

In complete shame, Billy tries his best to get in contact with the podcasters but they don't have any time for him now. For the second time within the space of twenty-four hours, Billy is shattered.

How did it get to this? he asks himself.

He starts to blame himself. If only I stayed home and didn't go for that stupid drink. Why do I care so much about her? She's just a girl. I am such a fuck-up. You idiot, say goodbye to any journalism career.

The more of these thoughts he had, the more he started to believe they were facts.

This not only affects Billy but also the people around him. His friends do not want to be anywhere near him because Billy often projects his anger on to others.

Billy starts losing everything around him – his sleep, his friends, his appetite and, most importantly, his sense of purpose.

He even cops a warning from work for rocking up late a few days in a row.

Billy just can't catch a break at the moment.

A few weeks go by, and Billy stumbles across a self-help book on the bookshelf. His mum reads self-help books all the time and she always seems to be in a good mood. Billy decides to give the book a go.

He smashes the book out in less than a week. He just can't put it down. It gives Billy the little bit of inspiration he needs to turn his life around.

Billy starts to change his daily routine. He begins by implementing a few daily tasks, like tidying up his room and doing ten minutes of meditation every morning. This helps him find some structure, brings awareness to his thoughts and boosts his overall mood.

After a couple of weeks of doing this, he starts including more of these positive routines into his life, including:

- Self-affirmations — he looks in the mirror every day and says to himself at least ten times, 'I love and approve of myself'. Billy even repeats this phrase to himself at different times throughout the day if he begins to find himself in a negative frame of mind.

- Setting daily goals — Billy invests in a weekly planner and hangs it up in his room. This allows him to prioritise and structure his day to assist him in achieving his daily goals.

- Writing what he is grateful for in a daily journal — before he goes to sleep, Billy writes down three things he is grateful for. He is grateful to have a close group of mates, a loving family and a purpose he is passionate about.

After implementing a simple routine that works for him, Billy is happier and more productive than he has been for a long time. He has learned to be kinder and more loving towards himself. That night was a traumatic experience for Billy but accepting he is not perfect and the mistakes he made are no reflection on the person he is has made the burden a little easier to handle.

Billy was his own worst critic and these routines helped him stop criticising himself. He would often talk himself down for not living up to the expectations he had of himself. By being more forgiving and using meditational practices as a gateway to presence, Billy has learned to see thoughts for what they are: thoughts. He is now more aware of his thoughts, often shifting his awareness away from them and back towards the present moment.

Billy is now pursuing his passion for journalism through creating his own YouTube channel while balancing his part-time job. In the first twelve months, he managed to gain 3,000 subscribers! He has the intention of turning YouTube into a full-time job one day.

Through believing in himself, changing his approach to life and being kinder to himself, Billy managed to turn his life around.

Even though this story is fiction, you may relate it to a situation you have been through. You do not need to find the perfect self-help book – just find inspiration in any way you can. This can be through talking to a friend or family member, doing some research on your feelings and thoughts, or finding a specialist. You are more capable of change than you think. If you have been interested in changing your life for some time now, all I ask is to just give it a go.

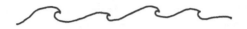

QUOTES & STORIES

WHAT DO OTHER PEOPLE THINK?

'We need never be ashamed of our tears.
CHARLES DICKENS, *Great Expectations*

'We need to cultivate the courage to be uncomfortable
and to teach the people around us how to accept
discomfort as a part of growth.'
BRENÉ BROWN, *Daring Greatly: How the Courage
to Be Vulnerable Transforms the Way We Live,
Love, Parent, and Lead*

'Breath is the finest gift of nature.
Be grateful for this wonderful gift.
AMIT RAY, *Beautify your Breath — Beautify your Life*

'I just give myself permission to suck.
I find this hugely liberating'
JOHN GREEN

'Do what you can, with what you've got, where you are.'
THEODORE ROOSEVELT

'Sometimes it takes a heartbreak to shake us awake and help us see we are worth so much more than we're settling for.'

MANDY HALE

'Every time your heart is broken, a doorway cracks open to a world full of new beginnings, new opportunities.'

PATTI ROBERTS

'Expose yourself to your deepest fear; after that, fear has no power, and the fear of freedom shrinks and vanishes. You are free.'

JIM MORRISON

'Courage is found in unlikely places.'

J.R.R. TOLKIEN

'The only way to make a spoilt machine work again is to break it down, work on its inner system and fix it again. Screw out the bolts of your life, examine and work on yourself, fix your life again and get going.'

ISRAELMORE AYIVOR

'Wanting to be someone else is a waste of who you are.'

KURT COBAIN

'Every saint has a past and every sinner has a future.'

OSCAR WILDE, *A Woman of No Importance*

'Time passes unhindered. When we make mistakes, we cannot turn the clock back and try again. All we can do is use the present well.'

DALAI LAMA

EGO

Sometimes losing is better than winning

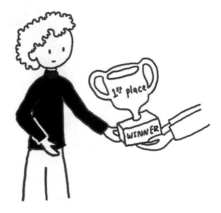

You have most likely said something to someone you care about that you wish you could take back.

This often happens with those who are close to us because we know so much about them. They become vulnerable to us, sharing personal things that have affected them in a negative way throughout their life. That gives us the power to really hurt them with our words, as we know exactly what will hit hardest.

The other person has the power of doing the same to us. We trust our loved ones to accept us for who we are. When someone close to us says something personal and hurtful, we take this criticism hard and it's a massive hit to our ego.

As we know, an argument can arise from anything. Depending on the moods of the people involved, the argument can become intense and can create a poisonous environment. When we get caught up in an argument, we become invested in trying to win the battle and making sure our point of view comes out on top. However, due to the hurtful things we can say, we may end up losing the war.

We can often have a mindset about our position in an argument: 'How are they not agreeing with me?', 'I am smarter than them, I am right!' or 'How would they know?'.

We don't get anything out of winning an argument. Sure, we might feel good for a short period of time afterwards, but it's not as if you win a prize: 'And the winner of the argument for March 20 goes to ... you! The prize today is a short hit of dopamine followed by the potential long-term feeling of regret and a loss of friends.'

We keep going and going until we hear those precious words — 'You were right.' These words do not often come as the other person in the argument is trying to achieve the same thing. Think back to all the arguments you have had; how often have you heard the other person say this to you?

You can often feel like you are more powerful for standing up for yourself and winning an argument. This can lead to seeking this power more and more. Try to detach yourself from power and winning. Look at taking the position of letting the person say what they have to say. Let them get it all out. Take a moment to analyse what they are saying and why they are saying it. Once you have analysed this, try to calmly either leave the argument, verbally or physically, or if the issue is important, try to resolve it in a way that is going to benefit everyone.

If you really do not care about winning, you can pretend you agree with them. Don't take this the wrong way — we should always look to be honest and, when someone is wrong, let them know, especially if their incorrect understanding has the potential to hurt them or others. However, for the sake of the relationship, agreeing often leads to an argument not taking place and to maintaining the friendship. Think of it as putting out a fire before it burns the house down. If the matter in question needs to be revisited, approach this person when they are calm and they should take the feedback positively.

If there is something you want to say, give it a day or two to make sure this is something important you want to get off your chest. This time will allow you to think over the importance of the issue and respond in a more measured way. We should try to never say or send anything to someone when we are in a negative mood (or drunk). You can always say it tomorrow when you have calmed down. if it truly needs to be said, you will remember it later and will be able to say it then — if you forget it, it doesn't matter.

As we discussed in a previous chapter, don't take everything personally. We need to question whether the confrontation is worth it. Stop yourself during an argument and ask: 'Is this confrontation worth winning?' and 'Is this confrontation worth losing or hurting a loved one?'

Refer to the chapter 'Make amends with someone you have done wrong by' to read more on a similar topic.

Don't let your ego take you away from who you truly are

Our ego can be perceived to be a false self. It is a mental construct that seeks approval from others and makes us live up to expectations — usually set by ourselves.

Ego shows up in multiple ways in our lives, including:

- being overly defensive to criticism and judgements
- being overly competitive
- not being happy with who we are and what we have
- having a need for materialistic things
- trying to please others.

The things that makes us feel threatened, ashamed and embarrassed have changed a lot over time: getting blamed for losing the game by your teammate, putting in the wrong measurements on a report sent to your boss, getting a B instead of an A on an exam or getting rejected by someone you asked out.

We think moments such as these will define us. We believe people will base their perception of us on the things we have done in our lives.

We forget why we are on this earth. We forget what came before us throughout time and what allowed us to live the lives we live today. World wars happened for crying out loud! Imagine if you were told you were going to be sent overseas to fight for your country. Would you be mentally ready for the uncertainty you would be facing? Could you leave your loved ones, risk your life and potentially see a mate in serious danger? Compared to this — is not getting your 'dream' job as harrowing or defining as it seems?

How can we control our ego and not allow it to take over our lives?

Be in the present moment. The ego cannot survive in

the present as it relies on past and future thinking. When something that happened in the past or something you wish could happen in the future is taking over your thoughts, take a mental step back. If you are thinking about a time when your ego took over, it might also help to ask yourself: 'What was my ego defending me from?', 'Was I insecure about something?' or 'Is there an underlying issue I am yet to resolve?' According to an article by Saul McLeod from Simply Psychology, the ego may look to use denial or rationalisation to avoid feelings of anxiety and depression. An example of this may include a smoker who denies smoking is bad for them.

Be where your two feet are and start noticing when and why your ego is taking over.

Labelling plays a large part in ego, too. By labelling someone who works at a fast-food restaurant as less than you, we only fuel our ego as we are putting ourselves above others. This person who works at Maccas is most likely working there part-time to pursue a greater dream, or it is the only job they can get at the moment and they are working their arse off to earn a living. Their work ethic deserves not only basic respect but to be held in high regard.

Be grateful for what you have as you have worked hard to get to where you are today. You have been through a lot in your life. Understand you have been through difficult moments and have come out on the other side a much stronger person. At times, your ego will look to bring you back to a negative mindset, fuelled by thoughts centred around insecurities and shame. When this happens, gently bring yourself back into the present moment and look to understand your ego without judging.

CHECK OUT

Jonathan Gravenor, 'The other side of ego' (TED Talk).

Saul McLeod, 'Defense Mechanisms' in Simply Psychology (web article).

Trying to be perfect

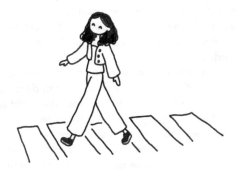

Something that links quite closely to the ego is working towards perfectionism. We want to be liked by everyone, be the best at everything and want to have no reason to be ridiculed ever.

Try not to work so hard to be liked because you will often lose and alienate more friends than you make.

Imperfection is what connects us as humans the most. Embracing and accepting people's imperfections allow us to feel comfortable and gives us a safe environment to express ourselves.

You may have experienced thoughts of doubt, insecurity and jealousy over certain aspects of your life. You may be envious of someone else or feel you are not worthy or good enough. This can often lead to negative thoughts, including: 'I wish I were tall', 'I wish I had the same hair as them', 'I should be the smartest in the class' or 'I should be dating that person'.

There is that voice in our head critiquing us on the decisions we make. If they have already happened, we may think, 'That was stupid, why did I do that?' Or, in regard to plans for the future we may think, 'This could come back to bite me, am I sure I made the right decision?' This voice in our head fuels us to try to be perfect and when we inevitably don't meet these sky-high standards, we cop a barrage of criticism from our inner critic, ourselves.

We can't say the voice in our head is wrong or wish it away; it will never leave. What we can do is accept it is there and also accept this is what the mind is wired to do. When these negative thoughts arise, acknowledge them without labelling or being emotionally attached to them. Think of these thoughts as cars passing by on the road. Once we have done this, we can focus on the present moment.

An effective way of rationalising these thoughts is to ask ourselves Socratic questions through cognitive restructuring as a part of cognitive behavioural therapy (CBT). This practice allows you to challenge and interpret your irrational thoughts in a more conscious way. A good example of this is as follows:

THERAPIST: Imagine that you are crossing the road and you believed that every car on the road was dangerous and could hit you. When you are crossing the road: what would go through your mind?

CLIENT: One of these cars could hit me.

THERAPIST: How would you feel?

CLIENT: Afraid and worried.

THERAPIST: What would you do?

CLIENT: I'd try my best to avoid the car, I probably wouldn't want to cross the road.

THERAPIST: Now imagine that you believed the majority of cars and drivers were safe: what would go through your mind?

CLIENT: I'd probably think that the cars would not hit me anymore (as long as I am being safe of course).

THERAPIST:	How would you feel?
CLIENT:	I would most likely feel safe. I would probably understand that most people on the roads are taking a safe approach to their driving
THERAPIST:	What would you do?
CLIENT:	I'd probably cross the road with little worries.
THERAPIST:	How does this make you perceive the links between your thoughts and feelings, and the links between your thoughts and actions?
CLIENT:	I guess that this proves that the way I think can have an impact on my feelings. I can also see how my feelings towards a particular situation/scenario can dictate how I respond to certain things. Is that the right answer?
Therapist:	It's not about being right, but rather about the conclusion you draw. What you just said — did you believe it to be true?
Client:	Well, yes, I can see that it's pretty believable — it is all pretty straight forward, isn't it?

This CBT scenario is inspired by *An Introduction to Cognitive Behaviour Therapy* by David Westbrook, Helen Kennerley and Joan Kirk.

We can see that through asking some seemingly simple questions, your thoughts can be interpreted in an entirely different way.

We allow ourselves to take a break from our thoughts when we think: 'I should be' or 'I wish for life to be better'. Be grateful for your life. If you are reading this, it is likely you have had better opportunities than others. You more than likely have a roof over your head, regularly eat three meals a day and have at least one reliable source of income. According to an article by Joseph Chamie for Yale University, it's estimated that at least 150 million people are homeless. However, about 1.6 billion, more than twenty per cent of the world's population, may lack adequate housing.

Next time you start having irrational thoughts about what your life should be like, start to question these thought patterns: 'Why am I thinking this way?', 'What is the evidence to say I am worse off than I should be?' or 'If I was someone else, how would I view my life?'

These thoughts are often common among people who overachieve. They are often incredibly organised, motivated, punctual and are committed to putting in the extra hours. These are positive traits for someone to possess. We do not want to be constantly lazy and lack motivation. However, these traits can be a negative, especially when we allow them to run our lives twenty-four hours a day.

When thinking about your life ambitions, it is important to know when to 'let go' for the benefit of your emotional health. Driving yourself into the ground is only going to make you more stressed when you either make a mistake or do not reach your goal.

I'm not saying to let go of your life ambitions completely, just take a break or a step back from them.

By letting go, we allow ourselves time to reflect on the good things we have done and the positive changes we have made to our lives. It also allows us to evaluate if we need to change anything further in order to make our lifestyle more sustainable.

You will often find this process actually allows us to have a healthier and more motivated lifestyle down the line.

Let go of the picture in your head of what or who you should be — the perfect house, the perfect partner, the perfect life. Take a step back and re-evaluate realistic expectations you have for the roles you play in your life, whether as a parent, mate or employee.

We may hear it over and over but we often don't take enough time to realise each person is completely different. You are a person like no other. You have your own thoughts, your own look, your own strengths and weaknesses and your own values. There is no one else like you and no one can take that away.

Love yourself unconditionally as often as you can. You are not perfect. You are going to make mistakes and that is fine because everyone makes mistakes. It comes with being a human being and not a robot.

CHECK OUT

Joseph Chamie, 'As cities grow, so do the numbers of homeless' in YaleGlobal Online (web article).

Elon Kline, 'This is why you are a perfectionist' (TED Talk)

Clark, G. I., & Egan, S. J. (2015). 'The Socratic Method in Cognitive Behavioural Therapy: A narrative review', in Cognitive Therapy and Research, 39, 6, 863–879

Peter McEvoy, 'Explainer: what is cognitive behaviour therapy?' in The Conversation (web article).

David Westbrook, Helen Kennerley, and Joan Kirk, *An Introduction to Cognitive Behaviour Therapy: Skills and Applications*.

Stop looking in the mirror so much

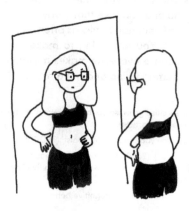

The mirror can often be an evil place for some people. We see ourselves—sometimes completely nude—and examine each part of our body.

Doing this fuels your ego as you are constantly trying to fix yourself in order to meet the expectations you have for the way you should look.

In most cases, it can lead to a lot of confidence issues.

You may be looking at the mirror to check up on a scab on your face from a pimple you grossly popped earlier that day. While you are doing this, you begin to dissect every aspect of your face—the bags under your eyes, your slightly crooked nose, a slight monobrow. You begin to feel incredibly self-conscious and start to have serious doubts over your appearance.

The thing we need to understand is that the mirror is not a true reflection of how we actually look to others. The lighting, reflections and colours, as well as the type of mirror you are using and the size of the mirror can all play a major part in the image we see looking back at us.

Do you ever notice pimples on your friend's face, their love handles, or their big nose?

The only person who is likely to care about your imperfections is you!

Try your best to stop obsessing about how you look. When you need to look in the mirror, spend no more than ten seconds there to make sure there isn't any food on your face or to quickly fix your hair.

By spending less time in front of the mirror, you will begin to find other, more meaningful, methods of self-validation. You will stop thinking about your imperfections and you will begin to like yourself for the way in which you handle yourself, rather than the way you appear to others.

Stop thinking about yourself and think of somebody else

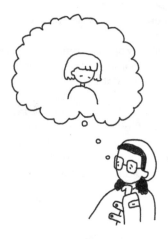

'Treat others the way you would like to be treated' is something you may have heard at school or work.

By being calm through mindfulness practices, including meditation, you are spreading contagious energy that encourages those closest to you to become a much calmer version of themselves.

Being kind and compassionate to others plays a large role in widening your circle of happiness. Offer your seat to someone on the train, buy some food or clothes for the homeless, volunteer for a charity event you are passionate about — it can even be as simple as paying for your mate's lunch. You will most likely feel a warm fuzzy feeling as you know you have brought a little bit of joy into somebody else's life.

People you help will be grateful for your kindness and it may even encourage them to do the same in their life.

It is believed that people who are kind are statistically more likely to live longer and less likely to suffer from heart disease. An article by Marta Zaraska of the BBC states that:

> Studies show, for instance, that volunteering correlates with a 24% lower risk of early death — about the same as eating six or more servings of fruits and vegetables each day, according to some studies. What's more, volunteers have a lower risk of high blood glucose, and a lower risk of the inflammation levels connected to heart disease. They also spend 38% fewer nights in hospitals than people who shy from involvement in charities.

By making a conscious effort to be kinder to others, you will become a nicer person in situations that you would never expect. Training the mind to be kind is vital, not only for your own wellbeing but for the world. By being kind, you are contributing to the optimistic vision of world peace.

CHECK OUT

Marta Zaraska, 'Why being kind to others is good for your health' in BBC Future (web article).

Failing is good

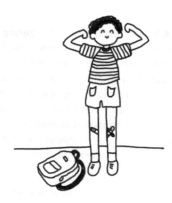

How many times have you gone home after a terrible day and just wanted to curl up in bed and hide away from the world?

If you look back on times like these, can you find ways in which you have grown since?

For example, say you went for a job interview for a role you always wanted. You did all the preparation in the world: role playing, company research, shopping for the interview clothes. You get there on the day, take a seat with the manager and completely crumble. You were asked questions you were not prepared for, the interviewer was intimidating and everything just seemed to be going against you.

Looking back on this is scary. Why would you want to relive that experience all over again?

Yes, you were unable to go through the interview easily at the time but you have now come out of that 'doomsday' scenario and are alive to tell the tale.

You also know what to expect when things go wrong. What can you do if you are faced with that scenario again?

For your next interview, you may look to implement mindfulness strategies to calm yourself down, or perhaps focus on other areas of your life to lessen the hype of the interview so you can walk in there more relaxed.

Of course, you can write this experience down in your journal to note how you can be better for the next time around.

These experiences are crucial for our character building as we can better understand that winning should never be taken for granted.

It is important to look back on our losses and find the positives in them. Knowing why we did wrong and where we can improve is vital for our growth as humans. Face your losses head on and learn from them as best you can.

P.S. It may be a good idea to bring back keeping score for all junior sporting competitions.

CHECK OUT

John C. Maxwell, *Failing Forward: Turning Mistakes Into Stepping Stones for Success.*

Say yes

✓ Say yes to that lunch with a co-worker.

✓ Say yes to that party.

✓ Say yes to that date.

✓ Say yes to that job interview.

✓ Say yes to helping your mate move house.

✓ Say yes to joining a new social sport team.

✓ Say yes to starting that new hobby.

✓ Say yes to speaking up at a work meeting.

✓ Say yes to having a productive day.

✓ Say yes to having a lazy day.

✓ Say yes to starting a conversation with that person you have always wanted to talk to.

✓ Say yes to starting that side hustle you have always thought about.

✓ Say yes to meditation.

✓ Say yes to loving yourself.

✓ Say yes to embracing your flaws or quirks.

✓ Say yes to working with and on your mental health.

✓ Say yes to growing and evolving.

✓ Say yes to living in the here and now.

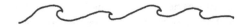

QUOTES & STORIES

WHAT DO OTHER PEOPLE THINK?

'If someone corrects you and you feel offended, then you have an ego problem.'

NOUMAN ALI KHAN

'Complaining is one of the ego's favorite strategies for strengthening itself.'

ECKHART TOLLE

'People call these things imperfections, but they're not, that's the good stuff. And then we get to choose who we let into our weird little worlds.'

MATT DAMON AND BEN AFFLECK, *Good Will Hunting*

'The truth is: Belonging starts with self-acceptance. Your level of belonging, in fact, can never be greater than your level of self-acceptance, because believing that you're enough is what gives you the courage to be authentic, vulnerable and imperfect.'

BRENÉ BROWN

If you can, help others; if you cannot do that, at least do not harm them.

DALAI LAMA

'Our greatness has always come from people who
expect nothing and take nothing for granted —
folks who work hard for what they have, then
reach back and help others after them.'

MICHELLE OBAMA

SIR JAMES DYSON

You would most likely or know of someone who owns a
Dyson vacuum. Sir Dyson made 5,126 failed prototypes
over the course of fifteen years before creating his
best-selling vacuum cleaner. According to Bloomberg,
Dyson is now worth approximately $27.3 billion. In 2002,
he founded the James Dyson Foundation to challenge
misconceptions about engineering and inspire the next
generation of design engineers.

WALT DISNEY

Next time you watch another Disney movie, just think
that these brilliant movies may have never been made
if Walt took the feedback of an editor the wrong way. He
was told he 'lacked imagination and had no good ideas'.
Disney is now regarded as one of the biggest companies
in the world with 116 movies as of April 2020.

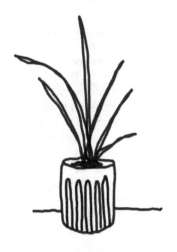

Wrap Up

Now that you have read through the book, take a moment to think about how it would be useful in your life. If you are drawing a blank, that's okay, just throw this book in the bin and forget it ever existed, but don't forget what I mentioned earlier — RECYCLE!

There are plenty of mindfulness and self-help resources out there that can give you great tips and tools to use towards living a happy and meaningful life, but only you can change your mindset to become more mindful. You are the one who needs to put the time and effort into yourself. If you are not willing to change, you will remain the same.

This will help you to respond rather than react when the shit hits the fan.

You can achieve and maintain this mindset through making sure your mindfulness practices are ingrained and are translated over into your daily life.

Plan out and set aside time in your day for mindfulness. Look to use this time for meditating, journal writing, a nature walk or just simply focusing on the breath. If it fits your routine and you see it adds value to your life, do it.

If you have a friend or family member who is interested in mindfulness, share mindfulness and growth ideas regularly. This will not only allow you to learn more about mindfulness but it will reinforce the practices and ideas you already know.

The world is a scary place at times. Your mind can be scary too. Work on being a better you every day and you will become more composed and aware of yourself in all life situations. Not only that, but you will also be able to respond to your thoughts, feelings and experiences with empathy, calmness and acceptance.

Acknowledgements

I would like to thank my family for all the support they have provided me with over the years. Thanks to the wonderful Amanda for your tireless work with editing this book. You were always available to do the little things (such as fixing references) and I am forever grateful. Thanks to Kellie for her quick and responsive editing of the book. Thanks to Nat and Jules for coming up with the incredible illustrations. These images capture the emotional tone of the book beautifully. Thanks to Tess for designing an incredible book. The book has its feel largely due to your awesome design work. Thanks to my mates for keeping my mind off the troubles of life and always making me laugh (you know who you are). Thanks to you for taking the time to read this book, this book would be nothing without you.

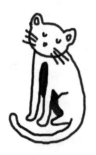

References

Better Health Channel, 'Panic Attack', https://www.betterhealth.vic.gov.au/health/conditionsandtreatments/panic-attack

Better Ideas, https://www.youtube.com/c/BetterIdeas

Beyond Blue, 'Panic Disorder, https://www.beyondblue.org.au/the-facts/anxiety/types-of-anxiety/panic-disorder

Smitha Bhandari (editor), 2019, 'What is Dopamine?' in WebMD, https://www.webmd.com/mental-health/what-is-dopamine

Body and Soul, 2017, 'Sally Fitzgibbons: "I won't start my day without it"', https://www.bodyandsoul.com.au/wellbeing/sally-fitzgibbons-i-wont-start-my-day-without-it/news-story/

Russell Brand, https://www.youtube.com/c/RussellBrand

Brené Brown, 2012, *Daring Greatly: How the Courage to Be Vulnerable Transforms the Way We Live, Love, Parent, and Lead*, Avery.

Brené Brown, 2010, *The Gifts of Imperfection*, Hazelden Publishing.

Charles Bukowski, 2007, *The Pleasures of the Damned*, Ecco.

Joseph Chamie, 2017, 'As cities grow, so do the numbers of homeless' in YaleGlobal Online, https://yaleglobal.yale.edu/content/cities-grow-so-do-numbers-homeless

The Chopra Well, 'Russell Brand's Story — Overcoming Addiction Through Yoga', https://www.youtube.com/watch?v=pE51o0izGFQ

Clark, G. I., & Egan, S. J. (2015). The Socratic Method in Cognitive Behavioural Therapy: A narrative review. *Cognitive Therapy and Research*, 39(6), 863–879. https://doi.org/10.1007/s10608-015-9707-3

James Clear, 'Warren Buffett's "2 List" Strategy: How to Maximize Your Focus and Master Your Priorities', https://jamesclear.com/buffett-focus

Cleveland Clinic, 2019, 'Irregular sleep habits linked to poor health', https://newsroom.clevelandclinic.org/2019/08/19/irregular-sleep-habits-linked-to-poor-health/

Sean Covey, 1998, *The 7 Habits of Highly Effective Teens*, Simon Schuster.

Stephen. R. Covey, 2004, *The 7 Habits of Highly Effective People*, Free Press.

Mihaly Csikszentmihalyi, 1998, *Finding Flow: The Psychology of Engagement with Everyday Life*, Basic Books.

Dalai Lama XIV, 1998, *The Art of Happiness*, Riverhead Hardcover.

David Lynch Foundation, 'Jerry Seinfeld talks Transcendental Meditation at David Lynch Foundation Gala', https://www.youtube.com/watch?v=uh7Yru3cHoA

The District Recovery Community, 'Top 10 Famous Addiction Recovery Stories', https://www.thedistrictrecovery.com/addiction-blog/top-10-famous-addiction-recovery-stories/

Michael Dulaney, 2018, 'Looking for an edge in sport? How mindfulness and meditation can boost performance' in *Mindfully* (ABC), https://www.abc.net.au/news/2018-09-15/mindfulness-meditation-sports-can-boost-performance/10215336

Caitlin Doughty, 2014, 'It's never too early to start thinking about your own death' in *Vox*, https://www.vox.com/2014/10/30/7047429/mortician-death-dying-caitlin-doughty

Encyclopedia Britannica, 'Sir James Dyson', https://www.britannica.com/biography/James-Dyson

Forbes, 2021, 'James Dyson', https://www.forbes.com/profile/james-dyson/

Gapminder, https://www.gapminder.org/

Héctor García and Francesc Miralles, 2017, *Ikigai: The Japanese Secret to a Long and Happy Life*. Penguin Random House.

Jonathan Gravenor, 'The other side of ego (TEDx)'.

Kory Grow, 2016, 'See Red Hot Chili Peppers Talk Special Pre-Show Rituals' in *Rolling Stone*, https://www.rollingstone.com/music/music-news/see-red-hot-chili-peppers-talk-special-pre-show-rituals-87012/

Rick Hanson, 2009, *Buddha's Brain: The Practical Neuroscience of Happiness, Love, and Wisdom*, New Harbinger Publications.

Jess Hardiman, 2017, 'Russell Brand is celebrating 15 years free from drugs and alcohol' in *Lad Bible* https://www.ladbible.com/entertainment/uk-celebrity-russell-brand-is-celebrating-15-years-free-from-drugs-and-alcohol-20171213

Headspace, https://www.headspace.com/

Headspace, 'Mindful death', https://www.headspace.com/articles/mindful-death

Health Direct, 'Dopamine', https://www.healthdirect.gov.au/dopamine

Health Direct, 'Mental health treatment plan', https://www.healthdirect. gov.au/mental-health-treatment-plan

Alana Horowitz, 2011, '15 people who were fired before they became filthy rich' in *Business Insider Australia*, https://www.businessinsider. com.au/15-people-who-were-fired-before-they-became-filthy-rich-2011-4

Hydro Coach, https://hydrocoach.com/

Gay Hendricks, 2012, *The First Rule of Ten*, Hay House Visions.

Anodea Judith, https://anodeajudith.com/

Anodea Judith, 2004, *Eastern Body, Western Mind: Psychology and the Chakra System as a Path to the Self*, Celestial Arts.

Jon Kabat-Zinn, 2013, *Full Catastrophe Living: Using the Wisdom of Your Body and Mind to Face Stress, Pain, and Illness*, Bantam.

Jon Kabat-Zinn, 2005, *Wherever You Go, There You Are: Mindfulness Meditation in Everyday Life*, Hachette Books.

Jordan Gaines Lewis, 2013, 'Why do we cry when we're happy?' in *Psychology Today*, https://www.psychologytoday.com/us/blog/brain-babble/201308/why-do-we-cry-when-were-happy

Kim, E. S., Hagan, K. A., Grodstein, F., DeMeo, D. L., De Vivo, I., & Kubzansky, L. D. (2017). Optimism and Cause-Specific Mortality: A Prospective Cohort Study. *American Journal of Epidemiology*, 185(1), 21–29. https://doi.org/10.1093/aje/kww182

Sebastian Kipman, 2021, '15 highly successful people who failed on their way to success' in Lifehack, https://www.lifehack.org/articles/productivity/15-highly-successful-people-who-failed-their-way-success.html

Elon Kline, 'This is why you are a perfectionist' (TEDx).

Ali Klinkenberg, 2016, 'Kelly Slater's guide to staying forever yung' in Stab Magazine, https://stabmag.com/style/kelly-slaters-guide-to-staying-forever-yung/

Marie Kondo, 2014, *The Life-Changing Magic of Tidying Up: The Japanese Art of Decluttering and Organizing*, Ten Speed Press.

Jack Kornfield, 2008, *Meditation for Beginners*, Sounds True.

Milan Kundera, 2009, *The Unbearable Lightness of Being*, Harper Perennial.

Ellen J. Langer, 1990, *Mindfulness*, Da Capo Lifelong Books.

Lucas, R. E., & Dyrenforth, P. S. (2006). Does the Existence of Social Relationships Matter for Subjective Well-Being? in *Self and relationships: Connecting intrapersonal and interpersonal processes* (pp. 254–273). The Guilford Press

Steve Maraboli, 2013, *Unapologetically You: Reflections on Life and the Human Experience*, A Better Today.

Madison Malone-Kircher, 2016, 'James Dyson on 5,126 vacuums that didn't work – and the one that finally did' in *New York Magazine*, https://nymag.com/vindicated/2016/11/james-dyson-on-5-126-vacuums-that-didnt-work-and-1-that-did.html

Mayo Clinic, 'Friendships: Enrich your life and improve your health', https://www.mayoclinic.org/healthy-lifestyle/adult-health/in-depth/friendships/art-20044860

John C. Maxwell, 2000, *Failing Forward: Turning Mistakes Into Stepping Stones for Success*, Thomas Nelson Inc.

Peter McEvoy, 2015, 'Explainer: what is cognitive behaviour therapy?' in The Conversation, https://theconversation.com/explainer-what-is-cognitive-behaviour-therapy-37351

Saul McLeod, 'Defense Mechanisms' in *Simply Psychology*, https://www.simplypsychology.org/defense-mechanisms.html

Mental Health Foundation Australia, https://mhfa.org.au/

Meredith, S. E., Juliano, L. M., Hughes, J. R., & Griffiths, R. R. (2013). Caffeine Use Disorder: A Comprehensive Review and Research Agenda. *Journal of Caffeine Research*, 3(3), 114–130. https://doi.org/10.1089/jcr.2013.0016

Mindworks, 'What is Zen meditation? Benefits & techniques' https://mindworks.org/blog/what-is-zen-meditation-benefits-techniques/

National Sleep Foundation, 2021, 'Three ways gadgets are keeping you awake' in *Sleep.org*, https://www.sleep.org/ways-technology-affects-sleep/

Freya North, 2011, *Chances*, Harper Collins.

Bailey Parnell, 'Is social media hurting your mental health?' (TEDx).

Ann Pietrangelo, 2019, 'How does dopamine affect the body?' in *Healthline*, https://www.healthline.com/health/dopamine-effects

Queensland Health, '10 weird things you might not know alcoholic drinks are doing to your body', https://www.health.qld.gov.au/news-events/news/10-weird-ways-alcohol-affects-your-body

Amit Ray, 2015, *Beautify your Breath — Beautify your Life*, Inner Light Publishers

Rich Roll, 'The Awakening of Russell Brand', Rich Roll Podcast, https://www.youtube.com/watch?v=qyRCQEum_vI

Hans Rosling, 'The best stats you've ever seen'.

Schwartz, J. 2016. Disconnect to connect: Emotional responses to loss of technology during Hurricane Sandy. In *Emotions, Technology, and Behaviors* (pp. 107-122). Academic Press

Robin Sharma, 2018, *The 5 AM Club: Own Your Morning, Elevate Your Life*, HarperCollins Publishers.

Minati Singh, 2014. Mood, food, and obesity. *Frontiers in Psychology*, 5, 925. https://doi.org/10.3389/fpsyg.2014.00925

Wendy Speake, 2020, *The 40-Day Social Media Fast: Exchange Your Online Distractions for Real-Life Devotion*, Baker Books.

Shunryū Suzuki, 1973, *Zen Mind, Beginner's Mind: Informal Talks on Zen Meditation and Practice*, Weatherhill.

Theosophical Webinars, 'Anodea Judith – Understanding your chakras', https://www.youtube.com/watch?v=yGj65ZFVVQU

Thích Nhat Hanh, 1988, *Being Peace*, Parallax Press.

Thrive Global, 'Kobe Bryant — The Power of Sleep & Meditation', https://www.youtube.com/watch?v=LdrVVJPIUK4

Eckhart Tolle, 2004, *The Power of Now: A Guide to Spiritual Enlightenment*, New World Library.

Jake Tyler, '"I'm fine" — learning to live with depression' (TEDx).

Matthew Walker, 2018, *Why We Sleep: The New Science of Sleep and Dreams*, Penguin.

Wang, Z., Mao, H., Li, Y. J., & Liu, F. (2017). Smile Big or Not? Effects of Smile Intensity on Perceptions of Warmth and Competence. *Journal of Consumer Research*, 43(5), 787–805. https://doi.org/10.1093/jcr/ucw062

David Westbrook, Helen Kennerley, and Joan Kirk, 2011, *An Introduction to Cognitive Behaviour Therapy: Skills and Applications*, Sage Publications Ltd.

Chris Woolston, 2020, 'Health benefits of friendship' in *HealthDay*, https://consumer.healthday.com/encyclopedia/emotional-health-17/psychology-and-mental-health-news-566/health-benefits-of-friendship-648397.html

Elizabeth Yuko, 2020, 'How to tell the difference between constructive criticism and bullying', https://lifehacker.com/how-to-tell-the-difference-between-constructive-critici-1844498083

Marta Zaraska, 2020, 'Why being kind to others is good for your health' in BBC Future, https://www.bbc.com/future/article/20201215-why-being-kind-to-others-is-good-for-your-health

Recommendations

Apps

Calm, https://www.calm.com/

Happify, https://www.happify.com/

Headspace, https://www.headspace.com/

Hydro Coach, https://hydrocoach.com/

Smiling Mind, https://www.smilingmind.com.au/

Books

Bonnie Badenoch, 2017, *The Heart of Trauma: Healing the Embodied Brain in the Context of Relationships*, W. W. Norton Company.

Brené Brown, 2012, *Daring Greatly: How the Courage to Be Vulnerable Transforms the Way We Live, Love, Parent, and Lead*, Avery.

Brené Brown, 2010, *The Gifts of Imperfection*, Hazelden Publishing.

Charles Bukowski, 2007, *The Pleasures of the Damned*, Ecco.

Dalai Lama XIV, 1998, *The Art of Happiness*, Riverhead Hardcover.

Dale Carnegie, 1998, *How to Win Friends & Influence People*, Gallery Books.

James Clear, 2018, *Atomic Habits: An Easy & Proven Way to Build Good Habits & Break Bad Ones*, Avery.

Sean Covey, 1998, *The 7 Habits of Highly Effective Teens*, Simon Schuster.

Stephen. R. Covey, 2004, *The 7 Habits of Highly Effective People*, Free Press.

Mihaly Csikszentmihalyi, 1998, *Finding Flow: The Psychology of Engagement with Everyday Life*, Basic Books.

Charles Duhigg, 2012, *The Power of Habit: Why We Do What We Do in Life and Business*, Random House.

Timothy Ferriss, 2007, *The 4-Hour Workweek*, Harmony Books.

Victor. E. Frankl, 2006, *Man's Search for Meaning*, Beacon Press.

Héctor García and Francesc Miralles, 2017, *Ikigai: The Japanese Secret to a Long and Happy Life*. Penguin Random House.

Seth Godin, 2007, *The Dip: A Little Book That Teaches You When to Quit*, Portfolio.

David Goggins, 2018, *Can't Hurt Me: Master Your Mind and Defy the Odds*, Lioncrest Publishing.

Matt Haig, 2019, *Notes on a Nervous Planet*, Penguin Life.

Rick Hanson, 2009, *Buddha's Brain: The Practical Neuroscience of Happiness, Love, and Wisdom*, New Harbinger Publications.

Dan Harris, 2014, *10% Happier: How I Tamed the Voice in My Head, Reduced Stress Without Losing My Edge, and Found Self-Help That Actually Works*, It Books.

Gay Hendricks, 2012, *The First Rule of Ten*, Hay House Visions.

Jesse Itzler, 2018, *Living with the Monks: What Turning Off My Phone Taught Me about Happiness, Gratitude, and Focus*, Center Street.

Phil Jackson, 2013, *Eleven Rings: The Soul of Success*, Penguin.

Anodea Judith, 2004, *Eastern Body, Western Mind: Psychology and the Chakra System as a Path to the Self*, Celestial Arts.

Jon Kabat-Zinn, 2013, *Full Catastrophe Living: Using the Wisdom of Your Body and Mind to Face Stress, Pain, and Illness*, Bantam.

Jon Kabat-Zinn, 2005, *Wherever You Go, There You Are: Mindfulness Meditation in Everyday Life*, Hachette Books.

Daniel Kahneman, 2011, *Thinking, Fast and Slow*, Penguin.

Marie Kondo, 2014, *The Life-Changing Magic of Tidying Up: The Japanese Art of Decluttering and Organizing*, Ten Speed Press.

Jack Kornfield, 2008, *Meditation for Beginners*, Sounds True.

Milan Kundera, 2009, *The Unbearable Lightness of Being*, Harper Perennial.

Ellen J. Langer, 1990, *Mindfulness*, Da Capo Lifelong Books.

Steve Maraboli, 2013, *Unapologetically You: Reflections on Life and the Human Experience*, A Better Today.

John C. Maxwell, 2000, *Failing Forward: Turning Mistakes Into Stepping Stones for Success*, Thomas Nelson Inc.

Freya North, 2011, *Chances*, Harper Collins.

Norman Vincent Peale, 2007, *The Power of Positive Thinking*, Fireside Books.

Jordan B. Peterson, 2018, *12 Rules for Life: An Antidote to Chaos*, Random House Canada.

Amit Ray, 2015, *Beautify your Breath — Beautify your Life*, Inner Light Publishers

Anthony Robbins, 1992, *Awaken the Giant Within: How to Take Immediate Control of Your Mental, Emotional, Physical and Financial Destiny!*, Simon Schuster.

Robin Sharma, 2018, *The 5 AM Club: Own Your Morning, Elevate Your Life*, HarperCollins Publishers.

Robin Sharma, 1999, *The Monk Who Sold His Ferrari: A Fable About Fulfilling Your Dreams and Reaching Your Destiny*, HarperOne.

Wendy Speake, 2020, *The 40-Day Social Media Fast: Exchange Your Online Distractions for Real-Life Devotion*, Baker Books.

Shunryū Suzuki, 1973, *Zen Mind, Beginner's Mind: Informal Talks on Zen Meditation and Practice*, Weatherhill.

Thích Nhat Hanh, 1999, *The Miracle of Mindfulness: An Introduction to the Practice of Meditation*, Beacon Press.

Thích Nhat Hanh, 1988, *Being Peace*, Parallax Press.

Eckhart Tolle, 2004, *The Power of Now: A Guide to Spiritual Enlightenment*, New World Library.

Eckhart Tolle, 2006, *A New Earth: Awakening to Your Life's Purpose*, Plume.

Brian Tracy, 2007, *Eat That Frog!: 21 Great Ways to Stop Procrastinating and Get More Done in Less Time*, Berrett-Koehler Publishers.

Hugh van Cuylenburg, 2019, *The Resilience Project: Finding Happiness through Gratitude, Empathy and Mindfulness*, Ebury Australia.

Matthew Walker, 2018, *Why We Sleep: The New Science of Sleep and Dreams*, Penguin.

David Westbrook, Helen Kennerley, and Joan Kirk, 2011, *An Introduction to Cognitive Behaviour Therapy: Skills and Applications*, Sage Publications Ltd.

Journal articles and academic texts

Clark, G. I., & Egan, S. J. (2015). The Socratic Method in Cognitive Behavioural Therapy: A narrative review. *Cognitive Therapy and Research*, 39(6), 863–879. https://doi.org/10.1007/s10608-015-9707-3

Kim, E. S., Hagan, K. A., Grodstein, F., DeMeo, D. L., De Vivo, I., & Kubzansky, L. D. (2017). Optimism and Cause-Specific Mortality: A Prospective Cohort Study. *American Journal of Epidemiology*, 185(1), 21–29. https://doi.org/10.1093/aje/kww182

Lucas, R. E., & Dyrenforth, P. S. (2006). Does the Existence of Social Relationships Matter for Subjective Well-Being? in *Self and relationships: Connecting intrapersonal and interpersonal processes* (pp. 254–273). The Guilford Press

Meredith, S. E., Juliano, L. M., Hughes, J. R., & Griffiths, R. R. (2013). Caffeine Use Disorder: A Comprehensive Review and Research Agenda. *Journal of Caffeine Research*, 3(3), 114–130. https://doi.org/10.1089/jcr.2013.0016

Schwartz, J. (2016). Disconnect to connect: Emotional responses to loss of technology during Hurricane Sandy. In *Emotions, Technology, and Behaviors* (pp. 107–122). Academic Press

Minati Singh, 2014. Mood, food, and obesity. Frontiers in *Psychology*, 5, 925. https://doi.org/10.3389/fpsyg.2014.00925

Wang, Z., Mao, H., Li, Y. J., & Liu, F. (2017). Smile Big or Not? Effects of Smile Intensity on Perceptions of Warmth and Competence. *Journal of Consumer Research*, 43(5), 787–805. https://doi.org/10.1093/jcr/ucw062

Podcasts

Russell Brand, *Under the Skin*, Luminary.

Dyl Buckey, *Dyl and Friends*.

Chloe Brotheridge, *The Calmer You Podcast*.

Kelly Exeter and Brooke McAlary, *Let it Be*.

Joe Rogan, *The Joe Rogan Experience*.

Jonathan Fields, *The Good Life Project*.

Jordan B. Peterson, *The Jordan B Peterson Podcast*.

Neel Kolhatkar and Jordan Shanks, *Neel + Jordan*.

Lynne Malcolm, *All in the Mind*, Australian Broadcasting Corporation.

Teresa Mckee, *A Mindful Moment*.

TED talks

These are available on the TED website at https://www.ted.com/ or, for TEDx talks, at https://www.youtube.com/user/TEDxTalks

Matt Abrahams, 'Speaking up without freaking out'. (TEDx)

Dr Kasim Al-Mashat, 'How mindfulness meditation redefines pain, happiness & satisfaction' (TEDx).

Richard Burnett, 'Mindfulness in Schools' (TEDx).

Joanne Davila, 'Skills for healthy romantic relationships' (TEDx).

Caroline Goyder, 'The surprising secret to speaking with confidence' (TEDx).

Jonathan Gravenor, 'The other side of ego (TEDx)'.

Johann Hari, 'This could be why you're depressed or anxious'.

Pico Iyer, 'The art of stillness'.

Elon Kline, 'This is why you are a perfectionist' (TEDx).

Kelly McGonigal, 'How to make stress your friend'.

Shannon Paige, 'Mindfulness and Healing' (TEDx).

Bailey Parnell, 'Is social media hurting your mental health?' (TEDx).

Preetha Ji, 'How to end stress, unhappiness and anxiety to live in a beautiful state' (TEDx).

Andy Puddicombe, 'All it takes is 10 mindful minutes'.

Olivia Remes, 'How to cope with anxiety'.

Olivia Remes, 'How to get rid of loneliness and become happy'.

Hans Rosling, 'The best stats you've ever seen'.

Zindel Segal, 'The mindful way through depression' (TEDx).

Max Strom, 'Breathe to heal' (TEDx).

Jake Tyler, '"I'm fine" — learning to live with depression' (TEDx).

Diana Winston, 'The Practice of mindfulness' (TEDx).

Web articles

Better Health Channel, 'Panic Attack', https://www.betterhealth.vic.gov.au/health/conditionsandtreatments/panic-attack

Smitha Bhandari (editor), 2019, 'What is Dopamine?' in *WebMD*, https://www.webmd.com/mental-health/what-is-dopamine

Beyond Blue, 'Panic Disorder, https://www.beyondblue.org.au/the-facts/anxiety/types-of-anxiety/panic-disorder

Body and Soul, 2017, 'Sally Fitzgibbons: "I won't start my day without it"', https://www.bodyandsoul.com.au/wellbeing/sally-fitzgibbons-i-wont-start-my-day-without-it/news-story/

Joseph Chamie, 2017, 'As cities grow, so do the numbers of homeless' in *YaleGlobal Online*, https://yaleglobal.yale.edu/content/cities-grow-so-do-numbers-homeless

James Clear, 'Warren Buffett's "2 List" Strategy: How to Maximize Your Focus and Master Your Priorities', https://jamesclear.com/buffett-focus

Cleveland Clinic, 2019, 'Irregular sleep habits linked to poor health', https://newsroom.clevelandclinic.org/2019/08/19/irregular-sleep-habits-linked-to-poor-health/

Caitlin Doughty, 2014, 'It's never too early to start thinking about your own death' in *Vox*, https://www.vox.com/2014/10/30/7047429/mortician-death-dying-caitlin-doughty

Encyclopedia Britannica, 'Sir James Dyson', https://www.britannica.com/biography/James-Dyson

Forbes, 2021, 'James Dyson', https://www.forbes.com/profile/james-dyson/

Jess Hardiman, 2017, 'Russell Brand is celebrating 15 years free from drugs and alcohol' in *Lad Bible* https://www.ladbible.com/entertainment/uk-celebrity-russell-brand-is-celebrating-15-years-free-from-drugs-and-alcohol-20171213

Headspace, 'Mindful death', https://www.headspace.com/articles/mindful-death

Health Direct, 'Dopamine', https://www.healthdirect.gov.au/dopamine

Health Direct, 'Mental health treatment plan', https://www.healthdirect.gov.au/mental-health-treatment-plan

The District Recovery Community, 'Top 10 Famous Addiction Recovery Stories', https://www.thedistrictrecovery.com/addiction-blog/top-10-famous-addiction-recovery-stories/

Michael Dulaney, 2018, 'Looking for an edge in sport? How mindfulness and meditation can boost performance' in *Mindfully* (ABC), https://www.abc.net.au/news/2018-09-15/mindfulness-meditation-sports-can-boost-performance/10215336

Jordan Gaines Lewis, 2013, 'Why do we cry when we're happy?' in *Psychology Today*, https://www.psychologytoday.com/us/blog/brain-babble/201308/why-do-we-cry-when-were-happy

Kory Grow, 2016, 'See Red Hot Chili Peppers Talk Special Pre-Show Rituals' in *Rolling Stone*, https://www.rollingstone.com/music/music-news/see-red-hot-chili-peppers-talk-special-pre-show-rituals-87012/

Alana Horowitz, 2011, '15 people who were fired before they became filthy rich' in *Business Insider Australia*, https://www.businessinsider.com.au/15-people-who-were-fired-before-they-became-filthy-rich-2011-4

Sebastian Kipman, 2021, '15 highly successful people who failed on their way to success' in *Lifehack*, https://www.lifehack.org/articles/productivity/15-highly-successful-people-who-failed-their-way-success.html

Ali Klinkenberg, 2016, 'Kelly Slater's guide to staying forever yung' in *Stab Magazine*, https://stabmag.com/style/kelly-slaters-guide-to-staying-forever-yung/

Madison Malone-Kircher, 2016, 'James Dyson on 5,126 vacuums that didn't work — and the one that finally did' in *New York Magazine*, https://nymag.com/vindicated/2016/11/james-dyson-on-5-126-vacuums-that-didnt-work-and-1-that-did.html

Mayo Clinic, 'Friendships: Enrich your life and improve your health', https://www.mayoclinic.org/healthy-lifestyle/adult-health/in-depth/friendships/art-20044860

Peter McEvoy, 2015, 'Explainer: what is cognitive behaviour therapy?' in *The Conversation*, https://theconversation.com/explainer-what-is-cognitive-behaviour-therapy-37351

Saul McLeod, 'Defense Mechanisms' in *Simply Psychology*, https://www.simplypsychology.org/defense-mechanisms.html

Mindworks, 'What is Zen meditation? Benefits & techniques' https://mindworks.org/blog/what-is-zen-meditation-benefits-techniques/

National Sleep Foundation, 2021, 'Three ways gadgets are keeping you awake' in Sleep.org, https://www.sleep.org/ways-technology-affects-sleep/

Ann Pietrangelo, 2019, 'How does dopamine affect the body?' in *Healthline*, https://www.healthline.com/health/dopamine-effects

Queensland Health, '10 weird things you might not know alcoholic drinks are doing to your body', https://www.health.qld.gov.au/news-events/news/10-weird-ways-alcohol-affects-your-body

Chris Woolston, 2020, 'Health benefits of friendship' in *HealthDay*, https://consumer.healthday.com/encyclopedia/emotional-health-17/psychology-and-mental-health-news-566/health-benefits-of-friendship-648397.html

Elizabeth Yuko, 2020, 'How to tell the difference between constructive criticism and bullying', https://lifehacker.com/how-to-tell-the-difference-between-constructive-critici-1844498083

Marta Zaraska, 2020, 'Why being kind to others is good for your health' in *BBC Future*, https://www.bbc.com/future/article/20201215-why-being-kind-to-others-is-good-for-your-health

Websites

Anodea Judith, https://anodeajudith.com/

Gapminder, https://www.gapminder.org/

Mental Health Foundation Australia, https://mhfa.org.au/

Mindful, https://www.mindful.org/

Outofstress.com, https://www.outofstress.com/

Positive Psychology, https://positivepsychology.com/

Australian Psychological Society, https://www.psychology.org.au/

The Resilience Project, https://theresilienceproject.com.au/

YouTube videos and channels

After Skool, https://www.youtube.com/c/AfterSkool

Better Ideas, https://www.youtube.com/c/BetterIdeas

The Chopra Well, 'Russell Brand's Story — Overcoming Addiction Through Yoga', https://www.youtube.com/watch?v=pE51o0izGFQ

Matt D'Avella, https://www.youtube.com/c/MattDAvella

David Lynch Foundation, 'Jerry Seinfeld talks Transcendental Meditation at David Lynch Foundation Gala', https://www.youtube.com/watch?v=uh7Yru3cHoA

Jordan Shanks, https://www.youtube.com/channel/UCaoxFlhy4oGz3EvkTGhWvkA/

Rich Roll, 'The Awakening of Russell Brand', Rich Roll Podcast, https://www.youtube.com/watch?v=qyRCQEum_vI

Russell Brand, https://www.youtube.com/c/RussellBrand

Theosophical Webinars, 'Anodea Judith — Understanding your chakras', https://www.youtube.com/watch?v=yGj65ZFVVQU

Thrive Global, 'Kobe Bryant — The Power of Sleep & Meditation', https://www.youtube.com/watch?v=LdrVVJPlUK4

CPSIA information can be obtained
at www.ICGtesting.com
Printed in the USA
BVHW041505070422
633677BV00013B/515